Managing Comple Healthcare

Managing Complexity in Healthcare introduces the ComEntEth (Complex Entropic Ethical) model as an integrated bio-medical and philosophical approach to understanding how people get things done in healthcare. Drawing on the complexity sciences, studies of entropy in living organisms and the ethics of Emmanuel Levinas, healthcare is theorised as energetic relational exchanges between people as entropic and ethical entities that unfold around a central attractor: Reduction in elevated entropy or suffering in patients.

Living entities are engaged in a continuous struggle against the tendency to produce entropy. From the cellular to the collective of human endeavours, the tendency of complex systems is to disorder and decay. Yet in the microactivity of healthcare enterprise, people resist this tendency by expending energy to create order and sustain life. Making sense of how this miraculous work is made possible is the foundation of this book.

Through practical examples – from analysis of practitioner burnout, rural and remote healthcare, the functioning of emergency departments, to government, social and institutional responses to the COVID-19 pandemic – this new integral philosophy provides practitioners, managers, policy designers and scholars an effective way to understand the dynamics of daily processes and practices that link the micro of everyday interactions with the macro-trends of healthcare.

Dr. Lesley Kuhn is a retired academic, Western Sydney University, Australia.

Dr. Kieran Le Plastrier is a family physician and Director of Medical Services at Blackall Hospital, Australia.

Routledge Focus on Business and Management

The fields of business and management have grown exponentially as areas of research and education. This growth presents challenges for readers trying to keep up with the latest important insights. *Routledge Focus on Business and Management* presents small books on big topics and how they intersect with the world of business research.

Individually, each title in the series provides coverage of a key academic topic, whilst collectively, the series forms a comprehensive collection across the business disciplines.

Organizations, Strategic Risk Management and Resilience
The Impact of Covid-19 on Tourism
Patrizia Gazzola, Enrica Pavione and Ilaria Pessina

Organizations and Complex Adaptive Systems
Masha Fidanboy

Managing Complexity in Healthcare
Lesley Kuhn and Kieran Le Plastrier

Work Organizational Reforms and Employment Relations in the Automotive Industry
American Employment Relations in Transition
Kenichi Shinohara

For more information about this series, please visit: www.routledge.com/Routledge-Focus-on-Business-and-Management/book-series/FBM

Managing Complexity in Healthcare

Lesley Kuhn and
Kieran Le Plastrier

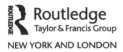

Routledge
Taylor & Francis Group

NEW YORK AND LONDON

First published 2023
by Routledge
605 Third Avenue, New York, NY 10158

and by Routledge
4 Park Square, Milton Park, Abingdon, Oxon, OX14 4RN

Routledge is an imprint of the Taylor & Francis Group, an informa business

© 2023 Lesley Kuhn and Kieran Le Plastrier

The right of Lesley Kuhn and Kieran Le Plastrier to be identified as authors of this work has been asserted in accordance with sections 77 and 78 of the Copyright, Designs and Patents Act 1988.

Library of Congress Cataloging-in-Publication Data
A catalog record for this book has been requested

ISBN: 978-1-032-05412-4 (hbk)
ISBN: 978-1-032-05415-5 (pbk)
ISBN: 978-1-003-19745-4 (ebk)

DOI: 10.4324/9781003197454

Typeset in Times New Roman
by Apex CoVantage, LLC

Each of us, at some time in our lives, will call out for help when suffering overwhelms our personal abilities to recover from the slings and arrows of fortune, and we will turn to health professionals for assistance. We dedicate this work to those professionals in healthcare who embody and enliven the ethical core of all meaningful action in the relief of our suffering, the knot of self-other responsibility from and within which all care arises. We recognise that they too can suffer, and hope that our work contributes in some small way to better making sense of the complexity that is healthcare, and their role in it. We hope our work might inspire new ways of thinking that support their efforts and improve the systems and processes through which societies organise the myriad relationships giving rise to the restoration and maintenance of good health.

Contents

1 Healthcare as Complex, Entropic and Ethical

Introduction

So, you're a physician in a busy hospital emergency department, and as you're introduced to your next patient you think 'How can I best find out what is really going on with this patient? What communication style should I adopt to have you tell me what I need to know to make a diagnosis?'

To define the case before you, you interpret the signs and symptoms presented by the patient and map out a course of action towards diagnosis and treatment. This involves additional information gathering, such as interviews with extended family, radiology and pathology, or another specialist review. It will be an iterative process as you test and re-test your hypothesis, all the while aware of the nurse manager's urgent reminder that you have this patient out of the emergency department within four hours.

Born of the uncertainty of the initial encounter and the models of working through the clinical problem, you arrive at your diagnosis and management, and ask yourself, 'Have we missed something? Are these medications worth it? How does this person understand what is going on?' So, you begin with some fluids and come back and check vital signs. Actually, you repeatedly return, re-examine and reassess.

This patient is one of 80 you will supervise treatment for in a shift (roughly a day). To do this well, you are dependent on staffing levels and expertise, effective working relationships between and with staff, patients and their carers, hospital administrators, availability of necessary technology and so on, and you are dependent upon the layout of the clinical environment so that you can physically get to each patient to check on them.

Importantly, aware of managing your cognitive load, you notice that your capacity to cope with huge amounts of stuff at once reduces when you are stressed and in survival mode. At those times, you pull back to become intensely focused on the patient in front of you, and you know that then you lose awareness of others and tend to become snappy with colleagues.

DOI: 10.4324/9781003197454-1

In popular culture, the emergency department (ED) has become a symbol of healthcare. It is for this reason that we chose to depict an ED as the opening vignette to this book. Based on a compilation of verbatim reflections of physicians, this vignette is intended to indicate something of the multitude of complex relationships that make the provision healthcare challenging.

Every day of the year, people experiencing illness or trauma and seeking care (the 'patient' in our shorthand terminology) and healthcare practitioners (registered health practitioners such as a physician, nurse, psychiatrist, physiotherapist podiatrist, chiropractor or other accredited health professionals) encounter each other at all hours of the day and night, in a diversity of dynamic and energetic environments – local medical practices, specialist clinics, allied health professional practices, hospital EDs and so on. Moments of loss and heartache unfold alongside triumph and banality, as humans and technology interact and engage to transform the experience of suffering towards its relief and the restoration of health and wellbeing. This is complexity in action.

Aside from appreciating the provision and practice of healthcare as exquisitely complex, we are interested in better understanding the nature of this complexity so that we might better understand what constitutes improvement.

Essentially, a theoretical explanation of the nature of healthcare, our intention in this book is to outline a complexity informed conceptualisation of healthcare and to thereby identify principles and practical implications, for improving patient experiences and health outcomes.

The ComEntEth (Complex Entropic Ethical) model of healthcare

Our fundamental postulate is that in *complex* phenomena, such as healthcare, complexity unfolds in *entropic* flows, under the influence of an *ethical* attractor.

We construe healthcare as *complex* because we understand that it is via multi-layered social interactions (such as between patients, practitioners, managers, administrators, policy makers) that healthcare exists. We say that in healthcare, 'complexity unfolds in *entropic* flows', because from a complexity perspective, these social interactions give rise to emergent collective behaviours, and because, characterised thermodynamically, these social interactions constitute energetic transactions and transformations (entropic flows). We describe these social interactions as *ethical* because we conceptualise the social interactions constituting healthcare, as based on, and organised in response to, an ethic of responsibility to relieve the suffering of others.

Thus, we propose the central attractor motivating and organising health-care activities as, *efforts to reduce elevated entropy or suffering in patients*, with this being achieved via ethically motivated reciprocal energetic inter-ventions between healthcare practitioner and patient. In this framing, improvement in healthcare occurs through reduction in development of entropy across the whole landscape of healthcare, including in patients and practitioners.

To explain the logic of this novel theoretical framing, we employ and integrate concepts from the complexity sciences, thermodynamics and the ethical thinking of Emmanuel Levinas. Firstly, we make use of the complexity sciences to present a conceptual framing of the structure of relations between stakeholders in healthcare. Secondly, we draw on the second principle (or law) of thermodynamics as it is understood to oper-ate in complex living organisms, to describe the structure of relations in terms of energetic transactions, transformations and management of entropy. Thirdly, we turn to the ethical thinking of Levinas to explain a relation of responsibility between the patient and healthcare practitioner as the impetus for enabling action within the structure of relations (why the person suffering illness/trauma turns to healthcare for help and why the practitioner cares). Bringing together complexity, entropy and ethics, we refer to our conceptualisation as the ComEntEth (Complex Entropic Ethical) model of healthcare.

In framing healthcare as complex, as unfolding through entropic exchanges and enlivened through an innate sense of responsibility towards the other, we offer a descriptive rather than prescriptive explanation. We are, in effect, offering a considered theorisation of 'how things are' rather than 'how they ought to be'.

Generative context

One of us (Le Plastrier) is a medical practitioner working in Australian public hospitals, who has long been interested in the factors that shape his and his colleagues' performance in the practice of medicine. The other of us (Kuhn) is a transdisciplinary thinker who, for more than 25 years, has been active in developing complexity thinking in philosophical and social inquiry. This book has its origins with the doctoral work undertaken by one of us (Le Plastrier) and supervised by the other (Kuhn).

An extensive review of healthcare research literature (Le Plastrier, 2019) revealed that while there are significant contributions and important insights offered within healthcare research into interactions between patients, practi-tioners and managers, an ontological, epistemological and axiological fram-ing was either assumed or incomplete.

The research team of the Norwegian interdisciplinary research project 'Causehealth, Causation, Complexity and Evidence in health Sciences' (Anjum, Copeland and Rocca, 2020) likewise critiques the lack of a secure philosophical grounding to healthcare and the way that philosophical assumptions motivating particular processes and practices have not been explicitly examined. They draw attention to the dominant influence of the bio-medical model of health and disease where all health complaints are assumed to be explained as physiological abnormalities rather than as containing biological, social and psychological elements, and to the way that care is often fragmentised, due to the compartmentalisation of healthcare into specialised medical disciplines.

This book represents an attempt to articulate a secure philosophical grounding for healthcare, and as such, it is concerned with applied philosophy. It is philosophical because it addresses fundamental assumptions concerning the nature of reality (ontological beliefs), the nature of knowledge (epistemological beliefs) and the role of values (axiological beliefs). It is applied because it explains how understanding healthcare as complex, entropic and ethical can enable and shape improved practice.

The perspective we bring to this undertaking is one that recognises, along with pragmatist philosopher, Richard Rorty, the folly of thinking 'that true beliefs are accurate representations of a pre-existent reality' (Rorty, 1999, p. 296). Rather, we are mindful that our beliefs about the world, our fundamental assumptions, determine what it is that we 'see' and give rise to strategies of action. As biologist and cybernetician Gregory Bateson reminds us, human knowing is 'bound within a net of epistemological and ontological premises which . . . become partially self-validating' (Bateson, 1972, p. 314).

We set out in this book a new way of conceptualising the complexity of healthcare that provides practitioners, managers and policy designers, an effective and novel way to easily identify links between macro manifestations and trends in healthcare, and the micro of everyday activities. It is expected that this novel ComEntEth model will assist practitioners, managers and policy designers to gain insight into the mechanisms by which the behaviour of departments, institutions and sectors arise, and facilitate the capacity of those involved to more constructively work together to improve the practice of healthcare.

History shows that humans have a predilection to explain experience and over time certain explanations have come to shape cultural, social and historical norms of understanding. Just as others have formed theories when they found themselves in the midst of certain life experiences (in a complex and ever-changing world) that they wanted to understand, this book presents our theorising of the processes and practices of healthcare. In accord with cultural historian Richard Tarnas's view that intellectual history is informed by 'tension and interplay – between critical rigor and the potential discovery of larger truths' (Tarnas, 1991, p. xiii), we do not see our theorising as indicative of understanding that is closer to the 'truth' of 'reality', but rather as useful to facilitating effective coordination of behaviour in healthcare.

A complexity perspective positions the human knower as ensconced within that which we observe, rather than as a separate independent observer. In this way, complex thinking construes human observing as participation in a relational universe where both the nature of the universe and human sense making (observing or knowing) are understood to be self-organising, dynamic and emergent. As Belgian Nobel Laureate Ilya Prigogine and colleague, Belgian philosopher Isobel Stengers, note: 'Whatever we call reality it is revealed to us only through an active construction in which we participate' (Prigogine and Stengers, 1984, p. 293).

In recognising the fundamental interdependence between the perceiver and perceived phenomenon, complex thought retains a sense of humility and requires that we build into our knowledge generation an epistemic level of awareness of the means by which our understanding develops. Our theorising, in effect, begins with 'Let us assume that . . .' and continues with a reminder: 'Don't forget that reality is changing, don't forget that something new can (and will) spring up' (Morin, 2008, p. 57). Thus, positioned between certainty and hope, we aim to provide useful indications for successful future action in healthcare.

Over the past 20 years, researchers have found value in viewing healthcare from the perspective of complexity (see, for example, Kuhn, 2002; Plesk and Greenhalgh, 2001; Sheill, Hawe and Gold, 2008; Sturmberg, 2019; Sweeney and Griffiths, 2002), where humans are conceived as 'composed of and operating within multiple interacting and self-adjusting systems (biochemical, cellular, physiological, psychological and social systems)' (Wilson, Holt and Greenhalgh, 2001, p. 685). The World Health Organization (WHO, 2006) similarly advocates that healthcare be understood as a complex system, 'in which there are so many interacting parts that it is difficult, if not impossible, to predict the behaviour of the system based on knowledge of its component parts' (WHO, 2006, p. 1). Our theoretical model of healthcare extends complexity based conceptions by explaining complex emergence in terms of entropic flows.

We understand healthcare as complex because it arises through multilayered social interactions between people, who learn and who are changed through these interactions.

Consider, for example, how dentistry, physiotherapy, podiatry, speech pathology, or other professional practices evolve. Whether as a private practice business or as part of the public sector, individual practices exist in a web of interactions, both contemporaneous and historical. Educational experiences, professional alliances, patient cohorts, client groups, research bodies, government policies and regulations, and the economic climate, all contribute to how healthcare practices function. Both professional practices and the individuals involved learn and are changed through these webs of interactions.

Other broader social interactions, such as contemporary dominant discourses (about, for example, what is important or how best to get things done) and dominant discursive styles of communication, contribute to how healthcare is manifest. Traditional as well as contemporary social media (such as Facebook and Twitter) strongly influence socio-political discourse and communication about healthcare related matters and influence public consciousness of what needs doing. Socio-political, social media-based influence on the practice of healthcare, while mostly devoid of an empirical base, can nudge contemporary dominant discourses towards accepting those views currently 'trending' on social media. So, ideas about what is acceptable in healthcare come to be those ideas that are socially approved, rather than those based on scientific and medical research.

The present prevalence of an economic rationalist perspective brought to most human activities also shapes healthcare, so that governments judge and are judged upon, how economically viable healthcare practices are under their remit. These factors, along with many others, have implications for matters such as funding policy to support education and research into particular areas of focus in healthcare.

In this book, we use theory to explain how thinking in terms of 'entropy' (a thermodynamic concept) provides a way of interrogating, and extending understanding, of the multi-layered social interactions and accommodations that transverse clinical, management, administration and policy interactions. As such, the book is intended for people who work for, or in, healthcare organisations and people who own, direct or have responsibility for managing healthcare processes and practices.

We interpret the term healthcare organisation in a deliberately broad way (drawing on anthropological and sociological interpretations), to describe complex patterns of human activity, that cohere around a common attractor of delivering physical and psychological healthcare (minimising entropy production). In our interpretation, healthcare organisations include hospitals, private clinics, medical research laboratories, health promotion and research institutions.

Arising through social interaction, the success of healthcare can be understood to depend on the human capacity to trust and cooperate with other people and to work together so as to improve patient experience and health outcomes. The model we posit intends to support trust and cooperation by providing a common means of explaining and describing activities across the diverse range of domains implicit in healthcare provision.

Positioning our theory

Karen Kitchener developed 'a three-level model of cognitive processing to account for complex monitoring when individuals are faced with ill-structured problems' (Kitchener, 1983, p. 222). We find this model useful for explaining the focus of our complexity informed conceptualisation of healthcare.

Kitchener describes personal epistemic development (development in how we understand, integrate, justify and apply knowledge) in terms of three, increasingly sophisticated, levels of cognitive processing (learning and thinking): Cognition (knowledge about a task or problem), metacognition (knowledge about which strategy to apply to a task or problem) and epistemic cognition (interpretation of the nature of the task or problem and the limits and certainty of knowing).

Rather than limit our engagement with Kitchener's model, to thinking about conceptions of ever more sophisticated levels of cognitive processing, we draw on these three levels to also think in terms of breadth of focus. We conceive Level One Focus as applied learning (rigorous disciplinary learning – biochemistry, pharmacology, genetics, pathology, biomedicine, anatomy, clinical learning, patient interviews, etc.) that attends to essential knowledge for engagement at the patient and healthcare practitioner interface.

Level Two Focus we think of as continuing an applied, patient/practitioner interface focus, but expanding this to explore and adapt the learning of Level One Focus, across different contexts. As healthcare involves inherent ambiguity and uncertainty in dealing with different patients in different contexts, practitioners necessarily engage a contextual perspective as they consider the ambiguities of diagnosis, treatment and outcome, patient response and so on.

We construe Level Three Focus as abstract, concerned with philosophical theorising; thinking about the nature and structure of reality (ontological beliefs), our knowing of it (epistemological beliefs) and the role of values (axiological beliefs). The conceptualisation of healthcare that we outline in this book is pitched at Level Three Focus. We propose a theoretical modelling of a structure of relations between stakeholders in healthcare (ontology), a framework for understanding this as energetic transactions and transformations (epistemology) and an ethical framing of why people who are suffering illness/trauma turn to healthcare for care, and why healthcare practitioners care (axiology).

In the following sections, we introduce the three major strands of our ComEntEth conceptualisation of healthcare.

Healthcare as complex

In our view, learning from the complexity sciences provides a way of approaching inquiry into complex phenomena (such as healthcare) that does justice to the complexity of life and experience. Complexity habits of thought, metaphors and vocabularies offer ways of identifying patterns and potentiality that are not bound to linear and reductionist assumptions and that assist in making sense of the complex messiness of life and experience (Kuhn, 2009, 2018).

Interpretations of particular findings and ideas from studies of complexity in nature, in concert with social and philosophical review and reflection, have over time evolved and coalesced into what is now recognised by many as an established 'complexity' paradigm (Johannessen and Kuhn, 2012; Kuhn, 2009, 2018; Morin, 2008). As a paradigm, complexity is concerned specifically with rigorous understanding of complex phenomena. By complex phenomena, we mean phenomena where there are multiple variables that evolve over time as they interact and influence one another and where the dynamic relationships give rise to emergent collective behaviours.

Healthcare fits this description of complex phenomena, as healthcare comprises multiple variables, including stakeholders (patients and their carers, healthcare practitioners, administrators, policy advisors) and health service organisations (general practice, hospitals, professional health clinics/ organisations) that evolve over time as they interact and influence one another and where the dynamic relationships between humans and technology give rise to emergent collective behaviours (such as cultural norms of a department, organisation or sector).

Complexity takes a radically relational view in conceiving how relationships between constituent parts give rise to collective behaviour and phenomena. People and organisations from this perspective can be thought of as 'contingent assemblages' that emerge from 'modes of relating' (Dillon, 2000, p. 9), or as Stacey puts it, 'complex responsive processes of relating' (Stacey, 2002/2003, p. 34). Complex phenomenon such as people, organisations and contexts, in this view, exist as processes of simultaneous order and disorder (Morin, 2008).

Framing healthcare as complex directs attention to the interrelating, self-organising, dynamic and emergent nature of the individuals, organisations, populations and environments involved. It emphasises contingency and inherent uncertainty, with individuals, collectives and context understood to emerge concurrently, so that what is known is constantly shifting and complete knowledge is not possible.

Viewing healthcare as complex in this way is useful because it:

* Acknowledges healthcare as irreducibly imbued with uncertainty – born of interactions between evolving factors or elements.
* Offers conceptual tools for discerning and identifying underlying patterns of order that provide depth of insight into processes and situations.
* Alerts us to potentiality, to possible future emergences by showing how interactions between multiple variables give rise to emergent collective behaviours.

Self-organisation, dynamism and emergence

Self-organisation, dynamism and emergence can be drawn on as basic organising principles of complexity. Self-organisation refers to the capacity of living entities (such as individual people, departments, institutions, sectors and so on), to evolve according to internal, evolving structures and principles (Kauffman, 1995). With living entities that self-organise, 'there is total equivalence between the phenomenal form and the principle of organisation' (Morin, 2008, p. 18). In other words, the form by which a living entity exists, is due to the internal organising principles of the entity.

Self-organisation accounts for how 'global order emerges without plan, program or blue print' (Stacey, 2012, p. 94), simply through local interactions between self-organising entities. This adaptive self-organising process can be thought of as 'self-eco-organising' (Morin, 2008), as it occurs within and in part constitutes a response to, an exterior environment that also self-organises:

> at the same time that the self-organising system detaches itself from the environment and distinguishes itself, by its autonomy and its individuality, it links itself ever more to the environment by increasing its openness and the exchange that accompanies all progress of complexity: it is self-eco-organising.
>
> (Morin, 2008, p. 19)

Dynamism describes how living entities have the capacity to respond to, and influence others, and the environment within which they are situated (Gleick, 1990; Kuhn, 2009). Dynamism is not merely reacting. Entities can learn to change their self-organising responses. For example, at a cellular level, brain cells 'constantly communicate electronically with one another and form and re-form new connections, moment by moment' (Doidge, 2015, p. xvii).

Emergence describes the capacity of living entities to display unexpected and novel properties and behaviours not previously observed. Emergence highlights how higher level order is created through networks of interacting self-organising agents (Johnson, 2001).

Individuals involved in healthcare (patients and their carers, practitioners, administrators, policy advisors) and healthcare organisations (general practice, hospitals, professional health clinics/institutions) exhibit key features of self-organising, dynamic and emergent entities. They each have their own purposes, dynamically respond to the environments within which they exist, choose what they take notice of, act in accord with their own internally evolving principles, and discover responses that their actions evoke, using this information to revise their organising schemas and behaviour (Stacey, Griffin and Shaw, 2000).

A complexity perspective highlights the critical importance of relationships, trust and communication. With healthcare organisational mores arising through interaction between self-organising entities (people and organisations), our relationships with others (both internal and external to the clinic/department/organisation) shape practice, and in turn, our relationships and sense of the trustworthiness of others, is dependent upon the nature and quality of our communication with them.

Continuing the process of translating and interpreting findings and ideas from studies of complexity in nature, we now introduce pertinent complexity metaphors, as conceptual tools, useful in better elucidating the structure of relations in healthcare.

Attractors

In complex phenomena, *attractors* function as an organising force that sustain behaviour (Lewin, 1999). Attractors limit movement and growth of entities as they evolve over time. Holding complex entities in particular patterns, attractors in the context of theorising human experience and sensemaking, may be conceptualised as energies that motivate. Identification of an attractor or attractor set assists an observer in understanding the drivers of particular behaviours of living entities (from individual people though to departments, institutions, sectors and so on).

A complexity perspective suggests that rather than viewing problems and solutions as attributable to singular cause and effect mechanisms between sets of deterministic interacting variables, it may be more fruitful to consider the mechanisms through which the behaviour of the whole entity is manifest. In other words, how the attractor (or attractor set) shapes the self-organisation, dynamic interactions and emergence of the stakeholders, and thus the particular manifestation of healthcare practice.

The opening vignette, in terms of this explanatory model, shows the activities of the physician, their colleagues, the patients, the patients' carers, and the administrators of the various departments (ED, radiology, pathology, etc.) as organised around care of the patient (maintenance and/or restoration of patient health). The physician, patients and carers, other healthcare practitioners (e.g. radiology and pathology staff) and administrative staff, are each understood to self-organise, as does the ED and the hospital within which it is situated. Each stakeholder is seen to dynamically interact with other stakeholders. It is through these manifold interactions that the particularities of the culture and practice of this ED are understood to emerge.

Phase space – phrase space

Simply stated, *phase space* describes a multi-dimensional plotting, over time, of all the possible states of a complex entity (Nolte, 2010). For example, H_2O in a phase space portrait would be shown as existing as ice, water or steam. Phase space plotting shows that although there are many possibilities, a complex entity typically occupies a minute proportion of its possible phase space.

Phrase space describes in an analogous way, how the habits of thought of individuals (healthcare practitioners, patients, administrators) and the taken for granted assumptions of various collectives (clinics, hospitals, national healthcare bodies) similarly depict self-imposed limits and restricted ranges of possibilities. Through phrase space, human collectives reinforce in their members, shared standards and ideas about 'what is' and 'what ought to be'. It can be useful to think in terms of phrase space, to assist in noticing and reflecting on preoccupations and habitual patterns of narrating events or responding to certain situations, and to thus foster insight into novel and useful possibilities and options.

The physician and patient, in the opening vignette, can be understood to bring to the encounter their own histories of existence within different phrase spaces. The physician's initial questions about how to most productively communicate with the patient reflect their awareness of the need to move beyond habitual, maybe medically oriented, ways of thinking and speaking, so as to have the patient provide pertinent information to assist in the diagnosis.

Communicative connectedness

Complexity directs attention to how human organisations are generated, sustained and changed through interactions between people. *Communicative connectedness* (Woog, 2004) refers to the quality and characteristics of interconnections between people. Communicative connectedness is critical in shaping forms of joint action, shared assumptions and future practice. In a hospital, for example, effective and frequent communication is critical to the safe and appropriate treatment of patients. Where communication is lacking, vital information can be lost and patient care mismanaged, with dire consequences.

In the opening vignette, the importance of communicative connectedness is recognised by the physician, in relation to not only the patient, but also the patient's carers and the wide variety of hospital staff upon whom they depend to provide critical and timely bio-medical interventions. Communicative connectedness between the patient and the physician, in the first instance, as well as between the physician and other ED and hospital staff, and the patient and other ED and hospital staff, is critical to the care delivered to the patient. Poor communication between the physician and patient might result in poor compliance with treatment. Poor communitive connectedness between the ED and various hospital departments could result in delayed or incorrect treatment.

Sensitive dependence on initial conditions

Often referred to as the butterfly effect, *sensitive dependence on initial conditions* (Gleick, 1990) highlights the dramatically disproportionate influence of initial conditions on shaping the emergence of complex phenomena. For example, an incorrect early diagnosis of a patient's condition can set in place a raft of consequential tests, treatments and health effects.

The initial conditions depicted in the opening vignette relate to the factors present in the initial interaction or clinical encounter, between the patient and physician: The causal factors leading to the patient's presentation at the ED; characteristics of the patient's physical, social and psychological presentation; the state of the physician (how tired, recent similar experiences, how they relate to the patient); the set-up of the space and ED resources, and so on. All of the factors present at this early stage can influence decisions about diagnosis and treatment, and can have significant and disproportionate influence upon the unfolding dynamics of the health status of the patient as well as the healthcare facility. For example, if the patient feels they have been treated initially in a timely and compassionate manner, their level of upset about their condition might not be exacerbated. Alternatively, a patient presenting with 'heartburn' who is not immediately attended to with expert care, might suffer severe consequences from missing a serious diagnosis like a heart attack, with implications for both the patient and ED dynamics.

Fractality

The term *fractal* refers to entities with look-alike features that are apparent across multiple scales of reference (Mandelbrot, 1977), such as the repeated branching of the circulatory, lymph or respiratory systems. Fractality can be usefully engaged to aid in recognition of situations where patterns of thinking and behaviour are replicated across individuals, departments, organisations and sectors. For example, an attitude that considers 'patient safety' as the most critical indicator of success might be seen to influence behaviour across all levels of healthcare.

In the opening vignette, fractality can be seen, for example, in management of access to resources to better enact responsibilities. This is seen with the physician in their patient consultation, where the physician rhetorically asks 'Are these medications worth it?'; in the ED, where there are protocols in place for use of various medical and time resources; in the hospital with respect to their management of resources in relation to a district perspective; and similarly, in national healthcare forums where policy decisions are made regarding resource distribution nationally.

Putting these understandings together, the practice of healthcare can be theorised to emerge through interactions between stakeholders, as self-organising, dynamic agents, in particular historical and social/cultural contexts. These interactions are conceived as unfolding around a major attractor: Care of the patient and maintenance and/or restoration of patient health. This framing suggests that adequate characterisation of the attractor (or attractor set) that guides healthcare practice is important, as it provides vital information about the types of interventions most likely to successfully nudge the enterprise towards optimal solutions. For example, interventions that are perceived to impede the capacity of the stakeholders to flexibly engage in pursuit of the restoration of health will be counterproductive.

The particularities of practices and processes in the service of care of the patient can be further illuminated and thus refined and improved by consideration of insights gained via employment of complexity metaphors. For example, though it is taken for granted a particular general practice is geared towards care of patients, reflection on communicative connectedness might reveal how care of patients is stymied by unclear guidelines to all staff (physicians, practice managers, practice nurses and reception staff), on correct responses to patients presenting to the practice with a cough and sore throat, during a pandemic, such as COVID-19.

Healthcare as management of entropy

Entropy is of central interest in thermodynamics, that branch of physics concerned with energetic transactions and transformations: How energy moves from one place to another and from one form to another. In thermodynamics, energetic transactions and transformations are understood to bring about the conversion of some energy to an unusable form. The term 'entropy' describes this unusable energy.

What follows is a non-mathematical explanation of entropy. We set out an in principle, stylised explanation of entropy, drawing on current formulations in physics, chemistry, biological thermodynamics, neurobiology, cybernetics and information theory. Our intention is to describe entropy in a way that is concise, comprehensible to a wide range of readers, and useful for engaging with our thesis, that in healthcare, energetic transactions and transformations, or entropic flow, is shaped by a central attractor: Reduction in elevation of entropy in people who are suffering illness or trauma.

The second principle of thermodynamics, understood to hold for all physical systems, is in effect a probability equation that expresses the tendency towards entropy (Morin, 2008). In essence, the second principle states that:

> The spontaneous evolution of an isolated system [a system without interaction with the rest of the universe] can never lead to a decrease of its entropy. . . . The entropy is always increasing as long as the system evolves.
>
> (Baranger, 2000)

This means that an isolated system, without help from its surrounding environment, will degrade over time as entropy increases. Simply put, an isolated system is 'incapable of putting its own affairs in order' (Baranger, 2000).

Biological thermodynamics, in being concerned with energetic transactions of complex living organisms, studies energy transfers in molecules or collections of molecules in open systems; living or organic entities that exchange both energy and matter with their environment or surroundings. Biological systems consist of processes of simultaneous order and disorder that are not isolated and that continuously receive 'help' (in Baranger's terms) to manage the degree of unusable energy (entropy).

Entropy was initially proposed as a mathematical concept that describes the quantum of random molecular disorder in an entity or a system unable to do work. Detailed and sophisticated conceptualisations of entropy have developed across a number of disciplines, including biology, cybernetics and information theory. Entropy has conceptually been extended to describe unusable energy as unavailable energy, disorder/dispersal, uncertainty and information loss in an entity or system (Coveney and Highfield, 1996; Hirsh, Mar and Peterson, 2012).

Entropy as disorder or disorganisation is associated with the pioneering work of Rudolf Clausius and Ludwig Boltzmann. In 1862, Clausius asserted that any thermodynamic process essentially consists of an 'alteration in some way or another of the arrangement of the constituent parts'. Boltzmann subsequently described these 'alterations in arrangement' in a mathematical, probabilistic formula. From this, entropy began to be referred to as a measure of disorder or disorganisation, with the amount of disorder/disorganisation linked to unusable or unavailable energy (Sharp and Matschinsky, 2015; Clausius, 1867).

Sometime later, in 1948, Claude Shannon introduced the concept of information entropy in his paper, 'A Mathematical Theory of Communication'. Shannon proposed a theory of communication, composed of three elements: Source of data, communication channel and receiver. In principle, Shannon entropy in information theory refers to a measure of how much information generated by a source is not received (Shannon, 1948). In information theory, entropy is associated not only with the level of fidelity of information received but also with 'uncertainty' or surprise, in terms of the information received.

More recently, in chemistry, in particular, entropy has been interpreted as a measure of energy dispersal or spread, at a particular temperature, rather than as a quantitative measure of disorder (Lambert, 2002). Proponents of this interpretation argue that 'From a molecular viewpoint all such entropy increases involve the dispersal of energy over a greater number, or a more readily accessible set, of microstates' (Lambert, 2002, p. 187).

Entropy can be drawn upon as an organising principle, to describe energetic flow (transactions and transformations) over time. Biological thermodynamics recognises that in living organisms there is a high degree of order, which is maintained by ongoing inputs of energy. Energy is expended in the processes involved in maintaining order (minimising entropy) and regeneration. However, this activity concomitantly contributes to increasing entropy (loss of useful energy) and to degeneration, thus requiring ongoing input of energy (Demirel, 2002; Katzir-Katchalsky, 1963; Prigogine, 1980). The health of humans (normal homeostasis) can be thought of as a complex process characterised by a high degree of biological variability, entropy and emergent order, with energetic inputs such as nutrition required to maintain normal homeostasis (Tuffin, 2016).

Viewing humans and healthcare organisations as complex entropic entities provides a way of making sense of inherently complex phenomena. Consideration of patient health and healthcare, from the perspective of entropic flow, enables identification of the dynamic capacity, interactions and longevity of the complex entity. If an entity is viewed as entropic, we can have expectations with regard to the past, present and future of the entity. We can ask, for example: 'Does the energetic input into the entity meet the energetic requirements of the entity?'

Literature on interoception (Demirel, 2002; Le Plastrier, 2019; Tuffin, 2016) suggests that human biological processes are exquisitely sensitive to changes in dynamic steady states that might indicate elevated entropy. Suffering can be conceived as a phenomenological experience of rapid significant elevation in entropy, and in this way, interventions to reduce and manage entropy in patients are understood as interventions to ameliorate suffering.

A person experiencing disease and trauma is a complex living organism experiencing rapid significant elevation in entropy (biological/psychological disorder/loss of energy), and thus, a threat to life. Healthcare recognises this interpretation of the person/patient and offers interventions to reduce entropy and energy loss. Healthcare practitioners offer melioration by fostering metabolism of free energy. That is, melioration is offered via interventions generated through the practitioner, that assist the patient in reversing or settling the entropy they are suffering. These interventions can be described as energetic transactions and transformations. The interventions offered may be as simple as a reassuring smile or explanation or administration of an intravenous antibiotic, or may constitute far more serious medical interventions.

Making sense of the critical constitutive parts and their relations, in terms of management of energetic transactions and transformations (entropic flows), we argue, is an effective way of identifying optimisation principles for improving patient experiences and health outcomes. We employ entropy as an analogy (rather than a precise measurement), to describe how uncertainty, unavailable energy, disorder and information loss manifests in and through healthcare stakeholder interactions and how levels of entropy might be appropriately minimised. Stated bluntly, we propose that optimisation in healthcare occurs through maximising dissipation in entropic flow (thus minimising entropy), in both patients and the humans who collectively constitute healthcare service organisations. This is because maximising dissipation of entropy supports the tendency of both humans and healthcare organisations in maintaining a steady state of least entropy production.

Bringing together complexity, self-organisation, dynamism, emergence, attractors and entropy, we can now further outline our explanatory model of the structure of relations in healthcare. We propose that energetic transactions and transformations between stakeholders (patients and their carers, healthcare practitioners, administration, policy advisors) in health services organisations (general practice, hospitals, professional health clinics) unfold around a central attractor: Reduction in elevated entropy (suffering) in patients, through the healthcare practitioner (physician, nurse, treating specialist, healthcare professional) offering interventions that reduce the development of entropy in the patient.

Placing the relationship between patients and healthcare practitioners as central to healthcare has applied implications for how healthcare is managed and strategies for improvement. For example, this model suggests that interventions that have a detrimental effect on the patient–practitioner relationship are likely to have profound detrimental non-linear effects on patient health and on the practice of healthcare. Interventions that place pressure on practitioners will likely be detrimental, as a practitioner feeling pressured, is experiencing raised levels of entropy and their capacity to hold and absorb the entropy expelled by the suffering patient will be impeded. Conversely, interventions that contribute to minimising entropy across all of the stakeholders can be understood to nudge the practice of healthcare towards more optimal outcomes.

Why healthcare cares: Emmanuel Levinas's ethics

Emmanuel Levinas (1905–1995) is a Lithuanian born, French philosopher whose major intellectual project was to develop 'a first philosophy', that is, a study of 'the first causes of things' and 'the nature of being'. Whereas previously, first philosophy denoted metaphysics and theology (Aristotle), or later, ontology (Heidegger), for Levinas, ethics precedes ontology (and epistemology). Levinas saw existence as fundamentally relational. He views relationships as necessary for knowing and asks what relationship to 'the other' (meaning other people) 'is necessary [an ethical question] in order for knowledge to be possible' (Ben-Ari and Strier, 2010, p. 8). So, a first philosophy in Levinas's view should be a study of the ethics of relationships:

> If the essence of philosophy consists in going back from all certainties towards a principle, if it lives from critique, the face of the other would be the starting point of philosophy.
>
> (Levinas, 1987a, p. 59)

Levinas's conceptualisation of our relationship with the other has come to be termed an 'ethics of responsibility'. According to Levinas, responsibility to the other is fundamental to human subjectivity. Rather than human subjectivity being defined by rationality or consciousness, Levinas sees subjectivity as constituted through responsibility: 'The subject is a responsibility before being an intentionality' (Levinas, 1987b, p. 134). For Levinas, 'it is of the highest importance to understand one's humanity through the humanity of others' (Ben-Ari and Strier, 2010, p. 5).

Levinas argues that as a consequence of being alive, people necessarily have a relationship with, and responsibility towards, the other. Levinas believed this sense of responsibility is known in the 'prehistory' of the ego so that the 'self is through and through a hostage' (Levinas, 1981, p. 117). For Levinas, this relationship of responsibility renders us 'both host and hostage' to the other. According to Levinas, seeing the face of another person reminds us of our implicit responsibility to the other: 'The face opens the primordial discourse whose first word is obligation' (Levinas, 1991, p. 201).

Levinas's main concern was to delineate an ethical explanation of the face to face relation with the other. For Levinas, 'The face resists possession, resists my powers' (Levinas, 1991, p. 197). He emphasised that it is important that we recognise the complete alterity of the other, that we see their dignity and worth as separate from our needs and evaluation of their qualities. Levinas stressed that we can never come to thoroughly know and understand another person; we can never absorb them into our own identity. He argued that when we meet another person, we step into another world, a world that is different from our own.

Levinas views our relationship with the other as making 'possible both the interiority of the self and a world held in common with others' (Young, 2021, para. 2). Levinas's philosophical assertion corresponds with the complexity sciences radically relational view of humans. Both Levinas and complexity emphasise how individuals come into being through relationship with others.

Levinas wrote extensively on suffering and compassion for the suffering of others. For Levinas, 'Suffering is surely a given in consciousness, a certain "psychological content", like the lived experience of colour, of sound, of contact, or like any sensation' (Levinas, 2003, p. 156). Felt suffering, made visible to other people, constitutes a call for assistance, an enactment of the precondition of responsibility for the other. As Levinas states:

> where ever a moan, a cry, a groan, or a sigh happen, there is the original call for aid, for curative help, for help from the other ego whose alterity, whose exteriority promises salvation.
>
> (Levinas, 2003, p. 158)

For Levinas, the clinical encounter, along with all human encounters, is a manifestation of, and only made possible by, the condition of responsibility within which humans exist. The 'moan', 'cry' or 'sigh' are expressions of suffering that 'call' us to action, to relieve the suffering of the other.

In our view, Levinas's conception of a relation of responsibility is an effective way of theorising the relationship that is enacted between the patient and healthcare practitioner. This relationship is understood as the impetus for why the patient turns to healthcare for help and why the practitioner cares. It is this relationship of responsibility that vitalises action within the structure of relations in healthcare.

As institutions, healthcare organisations are not capable of responding to a person's suffering. Rather it is the people involved who are capable of responding to distress and suffering.

Levinas's ethics of responsibility and his theorising of the experience of suffering provide an ethical basis to explain the energetic power of suffering. A rapid elevation in entropy within a person's biological processes signals disease or trauma, a potential for the loss of life. The person becomes conscious of discomfort or pain and may signal to others, by a cry or groan, that they are suffering. In terms of the Levinasian ethical knot of responsibility, when other people – such as healthcare practitioners – hear the cry or groan it elicits in them a desire to provide relief from suffering. From a biological thermodynamics perspective, we know that it is possible to recruit and administer non-random intentional energy into degrading processes or entities (such as the suffering person) to arrest and even reverse the entropic forces. In a clinical encounter, the medical practitioner is a critical part of the recruited interventional energy.

Healthcare institutions constitute organised processes of response to suffering. They bring together sophisticated technology and knowledgeable professionals to offer coordinated, non-random, energetic interventions into bodily and mental phenomena that are becoming more disordered, so as to support homeostatic processes and help restore a steady state and thereby relieve suffering.

In centralising and coordinating the collective efforts of humans to relieve suffering, healthcare institutions represent an economy of energetic expenditure by civilisations, to promote dissipation of entropy and thus increase the chance of recovery. The organising principle of the response to the suffering of the self and others can thus be characterised as an economy of energetic expenditure in terms of the second principle (law) of thermodynamics. The cry elicits a response that promotes mechanisms to assist in the dissipation of elevated entropy.

The opening vignette is set in a hospital ED, an institution that exists only through the provocation of suffering. The expert knowledge of the physician, and other healthcare practitioners, is focused on defining the case and mapping out a course of action towards diagnosis and treatment. The treatment is designed to promote dissipation of entropy and thus minimise suffering. The healthcare practitioners are working in an institution that has evolved out of a historical and collective recognition of responsibility to the other. The physician's intense focus on how to communicate with and treat the patient, and their ongoing concern to check, re-examine and reassess, can be explained through Levinas's conception of a relation of responsibility.

Thinking about Levinas's ethical framework as 'descriptive' rather than 'prescriptive', and his assertion that humans innately carry a predisposition to care for the other, it is interesting to ponder occasions when care for another is not observed. What factors might give rise to such occasions? Three come to mind in reflecting on the opening vignette. The first, is that through excessive responsibility, cognitive load and busyness, we might not 'see' the other, as other, but rather as 'objects', instrumental to our requirements, or as a background to our activities. Supervising 80 patients in an ED in a shift, inadequate staffing levels, ineffective working relationships, unavailability of necessary technology, an unwieldy physical layout of the clinical environment, all might contribute to not properly relating to other people.

Secondly, de-humanising the other person would render them as no longer thought of as the other. An obvious example of this is in warfare. However, there is a potential for such de-humanising to occur in the practice of healthcare. For example, patients can be viewed only as a particular illness/trauma or bodily part, rather than as a suffering person. Again, it might be through excessive busyness and stress that healthcare practitioners inadvertently seek to manage their own cognitive overload and increase in production of entropy, by focusing on the trauma rather than the whole person or on the personhood of colleagues.

Three, when we presume to completely know the other, based on our own knowledge and experience, we reduce them to our own limited frames of knowing and being, rather than respect the other person's alterity. In healthcare, this might mean our attending to the patient becomes more about our own projections or interventions that we habitually offer, and less about what the person requires. Providing bio-medical care, based on expert knowledge and experience, while recognising that the suffering person is radically different from myself, requires an attitude of openness and humility. Healthcare practice constitutes situations where the relationship is unequal with weakness and dependency on the one side, and power, expertise and patronage on the other. This might contribute to reducing in healthcare practitioners, a sense of openness and humility towards the other.

Improvement in healthcare as reduction in development of entropy

In the preceding discussion of our ComEntEth theoretical framing of healthcare, we elaborated our thinking in support of our fundamental postulate, that 'in complex phenomena such as healthcare, complexity unfolds in entropic flows under the influence of ethical attractors', and corollary, that improvement in healthcare occurs through reduction in development of entropy.

Based on this framing, the logic of the argument outlined in this book is that:

- Humans, as complex entropic entities, seek to manage internal entropy as they dynamically self-organise.
- Suffering in humans constitutes a phenomenological experience of significant elevation in entropy.
- Humans can seek help from others (such as healthcare practitioners) to reduce suffering or elevated entropy.
- Healthcare practitioners seek to ameliorate suffering by offering interventions that reduce the development of entropy in the person experiencing illness/trauma (patient).
- Interaction between the patient and healthcare practitioner (the clinical encounter) is central to the capacity of healthcare to reduce entropy.
- The principle of seeking to reduce the development of entropy (suffering) holds as the *raison d'etre* across all activities within healthcare (including health promotion as a strategy to prevent the development of elevated entropy).
- Reduction of entropy across the multi-layered interactions through which healthcare emerges significantly supports the capacity of practitioners to reduce the patient's elevated entropy, and to engage in health promotion activities.

In sum, we conceptualise healthcare as constituted by energetic relational exchanges between, in the language of complexity, self-organising, dynamic and emergent entities. These energetic relational exchanges unfold around a central attractor, reduction in suffering or development of elevated entropy in patients, through the healthcare practitioner offering appropriate energetic interventions. This process, in Levinas's conceptualisation, is made possible through humans being in a relationship of responsibility and care for one another. Under the logic of our ComEntEth model, both bio-medicine and relational ethics are implicated in preventing or resolving the patient's entropic elevation. The relational exchanges, in thermodynamic terms, constitute energetic transactions and transformations, that inevitably, generate entropy. Entropic reverberations across healthcare organisations are therefore to be expected. We argue that through noticing entropic levels, powerful insights can be gained into how people are collectively organising (relating) to 'get things done' in healthcare. In our framing, indicators for improvement can be gleaned by examining the nature and quality of relationships. Do they facilitate an increase or decrease in entropy?

Structure of the book

The following chapters advance our ComEntEth conceptualisation of healthcare. We identify principles and practices for minimising entropy levels within the patient–practitioner relationship and across stakeholders and healthcare organisations.

In Chapter 2, we elaborate a bio-medical explanation of suffering as elevation in entropy (biological/psychological disorganisation), and show how healthcare is concerned ultimately, with management of entropy. We explain (1) how conceptualising complex interactions and emergence as entropic transactions and transformations, offers a unified way of perceiving trauma and illness, alleviating treatments, and the multitude of complex relationships implicated in healthcare and (2) how bio-medicine and organisational dynamics are conjoined in efforts to manage elevated entropy (suffering). The chapter concludes with a practical illustration of the potential for our ComEntEth conceptualisation of healthcare to facilitate beneficial insights that lead to improvements in practice.

In Chapter 3, we theorise how improvement in healthcare occurs by minimising entropy development in healthcare organisations. We explore how the multiple social interactions through which habitual processes and practices of getting things done, increase or minimise entropy production in individuals and collectives. Principles and practices that minimise entropy production are discussed with reference to major themes in healthcare and organisation studies literature. Through analysis of two vignettes, we demonstrate how conceptualising healthcare as complex, entropic and ethical can stimulate new insights that can lead to improvement in practice.

In Chapter 4, we demonstrate the utility of studying government, social and organisational responses, from the perspective of our ComEntEth model, to make sense of why and how the world has evolved different outcomes in response to the shared crisis of the SARS-CoV-2 pandemic. We explore how pandemics induce rapid increase in entropy that threaten the viability of individuals, healthcare organisations and the broader societal contexts within which they are situated. In conclusion, we propose principles and practices for optimisation of strategic responses to pandemics.

In Chapter 5, we summarise the benefits of understanding healthcare as a complex phenomenon, wherein complexity unfolds in entropic flows, via responsive processes of relating, under the influence of an ethical attractor. We offer suggestions for further exploring how utilisation of our ComEntEth model can aid understanding of the relational exchanges that give rise to healthcare processes and practices.

References

Anjum, R. L., Copeland, S. and Rocca, E. (2020) *Rethinking Causality, Complexity and Evidence for the Unique Patient*. Switzerland: Springer.

Baranger, M. (2000) *Chaos, Complexity, and Entropy: A Physics Talk for Non-Physicists*. Cambridge, MA: New England Complex Systems Institute. https://necsi.edu/chaos-complexity-and-entropy.

Bateson, G. (1972) *Steps to an Ecology of Mind*. San Francisco: Chandler Publications.

Ben-Ari, A. and Strier, R. (2010) 'Rethinking Cultural Competence: What Can We Learn From Levinas?'. *British Journal of Social Work*. 2010:1–13.

Clausius, R. (1867) *The Mechanical Theory of Heat, With Its Applications to the Steam Engine and to the Physical Properties of Bodies* (T. Archer Hirst, Ed). London: J. Van Voorst.

Coveney, P. and Highfield, R. (1996) *Frontiers of Complexity*. London: Faber and Faber.

Demirel, Y. (2002) *Nonequilibrium Thermodynamics: Transport and Rate Processes in Physical and Biological Systems*. Blacksburg: Elsevier Science.

Dillon, M. (2000) 'Poststructuralism, Complexity and Poetics'. *Theory, Culture & Society*. 17(5):1–26.

Doidge, N. (2015) *The Brain's Way of Healing*. Victoria: Scribe.

Gleick, J. (1990) *Chaos: Making a New Science*. London: Cardinal.

Hirsh, J. B., Mar, R. A. and Peterson, J. B. (2012) 'Psychological Entropy: A Framework for Understanding Uncertainty-Related Anxiety'. *Psychological Review*. 119(20):304–320.

Johannessen, S. O. and Kuhn, L. (Eds) (2012) 'Introduction: Ways of Thinking About Complexity'. *Complexity in Organisation Studies* (Vol. 1). London: Sage.

Johnson, S. (2001) *Emergence*. London: Allen Lane The Penguin Press.

Katzir-Katchalsky, A. (1963) 'Non-Equilibrium Thermodynamics'. *International Science Tech*. 1963;43–49.

Kauffman, S. (1995) *At Home in the Universe: The Search for the Laws of Self-Organisations and Complexity*. Oxford: Oxford University Press.

Kitchener, K. S. (1983) 'Cognition, Metacognition and Epistemic Cognition: A Three Level Model of Cognitive Processing'. *Human Development*. 26:222–232.

Kuhn, L. (2002) 'Health Promotion and Complexity Theory: An Approach for the 21st Century'. Dimitrov, V. and Naess, T. (Eds) *Health Ecology: Learning to Cope with Complex Realities*. Asker: NaKuHel. Pp. 135–146.

Kuhn, L. (2009) *Adventures in Complexity for Organisations Near the Edge of Chaos*. Axminster: Triarchy Press.

Kuhn, L. (2018) 'Complexity Informed Social Research: From Complexity Concepts to Creative Applications'. Mitleton-Kelly, E., Paraskevas, A. and Day, C. (Eds) *Handbook of Research Methods in Complexity Science*. Cheltenham: Edward Elgar Publishing.

Lambert, F. L. (2002) 'Disorder: A Cracked Crutch for Supporting Entropy Discussions'. *Journal of Chemical Education*. 79(2):187.

Le Plastrier, K. (2019) 'The Entropy of Suffering: An Inquiry Into the Consequences of the 4-Hour Rule for the Patient–Doctor Relationship in Australian Public Hospitals'. Doctoral thesis, Western Sydney University.

Levinas, E. (1974/1981) *Otherwise Than Being or Beyond Essence* (A. Lingis, Trans). Pittsburgh: Duquesne University Press.

Levinas, E. (1987a) 'Philosophy and the Idea of Infinity'. *Collected Philosophical Papers* (A. Lingis, Trans). New York: Springer.

Levinas, E. (1987b) 'Humanism and Anarchy'. *Collected Philosophical Papers* (A. Lingis, Trans). New York: Springer.

Levinas, E. (1961/1991) *Totality and Infinity: An Essay on Exteriority* (A. Lingis, Trans). Dordrecht: Kluwer Academic Publishers.

Levinas, E. (2003) 'Useless Suffering'. Bernasconi, R. and Wood, D. (Eds) *The Provocation of Levinas: Rethinking the Other* (R. Cohen, Trans). London: Routledge.

Lewin, R. (1999) 'Complexity: The Science, Its Vocabulary, and Its Relation to Organisations'. *Emergence*. 1(1):110–126.

Mandelbrot, B. (1977) *The Fractal Geometry of Nature*. New York: Freeman.

Morin, E. (2008) *On Complexity* (R. Postel and M. Kelly, Trans). NJ: Hampton Press.

Nolte, D. (2010) 'The Tangled Tale of Phase Space'. *Physics Today*. 63(40):10. doi:1063/1.3397041

Plesk, P. E. and Greenhalgh, T. (2001) 'Complexity Science: The Challenge of Complexity in Health Care'. *British Medical Journal*. 323:625–628.

Prigogine, I. (1980) *From Being to Becoming: Time and Complexity in the Physical Sciences*. San Francisco: Freeman.

Prigogine, I. and Stengers, I. (1984) *Order Out of Chaos*. New York: bantam Books.

Rorty, R. (1999) *Philosophy and Social Hope*. London: Penguin Books.

Shannon, C. E. (1948) 'A Mathematical Theory of Communication'. *Bell System Technology Journal*. 27(3):379–423.

Sharp, K. and Matschinsky, F. (2015) 'Translation of Ludwig Boltzmann's Paper "On the Relationship between the Second Fundamental Theorem of the Mechanical Theory of Heat and Probability Calculations Regarding the Conditions for Thermal Equilibrium" Sitzungberichte der Kaiserlichen Akademie der Wissenschaften. Mathematisch-Naturwissen Class. Abt. II, LXXVI 1877, pp. 373–435 (Wien. Ber. 1877, 76:373–435. Reprinted in Wiss. Abhandlungen, Vol. II, reprint 42, p. 164–223, Barth, Leipzig, 1909'. *Entropy*. 2015(17):1971–2009. doi:10.3390/e17041971

Sheill, A., Hawe, P. and Gold, L. (2008) 'Complex Interventions or Complex Systems? Implications for Health Economic Evaluation'. *British Medical Journal*. 336:1281–1283.

Stacey, R. D. (2002/2003) 'Organisations as Complex Responsive Processes of Relating'. *Journal of Innovative Management*. 8(2):27–39.

Stacey, R. D. (2012) 'Comment on Debate Article: Coaching Psychology Coming of Age: The Challenges We Face in the Messy World of Complexity'. *International Coaching Psychology Review*. 7(1):91–95.

Stacey, R. D., Griffin, D. and Shaw, P. (2000) *Complexity and Management*. London: Routledge.

Sturmberg, J. (Ed) (2019) *Embracing Complexity in Health: The Transformation of Science, Practice, and Policy*. New York: Springer.

Sweeney, K. and Griffiths, F. (2002) *Complexity and Healthcare: An Introduction*. Oxford: Radcliffe Medical Press.

Tarnas, R. (1991) *The Passion of the Western Mind*. New York: Ballantine Books.

Tuffin, R. (2016) 'Implications of Complexity Theory for Clinical Practice and Healthcare Organization'. *BJA Education*. 16(10):349–352.

Wilson, T., Holt, T. A. and Greenhalgh, T. (2001) 'Complexity Science: Complexity and Clinical care'. *British Medical Journal*. 323(7314):685–688.

Woog, R. (2004) 'The Knowing of Knowledge'. Australian Training Authority. *Working and Learning in Vocational Education and Training in the Knowledge Era*. www.flexiblelearning.net.au/projects/resources/PDFutureF.doc.

World Health Organization (WHO) (2006) 'To Err Is Human'. *Patient Safety*. DOC:1.4.

2 Reducing Entropy in Patients as the Essence of Healthcare

Introduction

As outlined in Chapter 1, complex biological entities are engaged in a continuous struggle against the tendency to produce entropy. In this chapter, we elaborate our explanation of how healthcare is implicated in this struggle against entropy production. We recognise that just as this struggle is fundamental to the bodily-psychological processes of individual humans, it is fundamental to social life, as humans interact with one another. In finessing our explanation of healthcare as being concerned ultimately, with reducing elevated entropy in the patient, we describe how this is achieved by interaction between the patient and healthcare practitioner, positioned as they are, within a web of multi-layered social interactions.

A practical benefit of explaining complex interactions and emergence in terms of entropic transactions and transformations is that it offers a unified way of perceiving trauma and illness, alleviating treatments, and the multitude of complex relationships implicated in healthcare. Furthermore, conceptualising healthcare processes and practices as entropic exchanges highlights interdependencies and reciprocality between bio-medicine and organisational dynamics, and shows how these are conjoined by a shared attractor, namely, efforts to manage elevated entropy (suffering).

In complex entities, such as healthcare, self-organisation, dynamism and emergence are conceptualised as unfolding around an attractor or attractor set, which functions as a major organising force. This is expressed in our 'Complex Entropic Ethical' (ComEntEth) model. Our thesis is that the major organising force (attractor) directing healthcare processes and practices is commitment to reduce rapid development of entropy (suffering). Suffering, or elevation in entropy, in this sense, is understood as a causal power that activates restorative processes, from within the internal biological processes of an individual, through to healthcare organisations.

DOI: 10.4324/9781003197454-2

In thermodynamics, the historically correct descriptor, for what in complexity might be referred to as multiple interacting variables or 'whole-parts', is 'system'. So, in setting out a thermodynamic explanation of the role of entropy in suffering we use this term. The term 'system' in thermodynamics refers to the particular item or collection of items being studied (such as a particular cell, or bodily system, for example, the endocrine system), and all that is not included in the system, is referred to as the 'surroundings' or 'environment'. When we refer to reduction or dissipation of entropy, we are commenting on how this occurs within the whole-part or system under review. The concept of dissipation of entropy relates back to Ilya Prigogine's coining of the term 'dissipative structures' to describe the means by which complex systems manage energy transfers and transformations to create increased order and so maintain life (Prigogine and Lefever, 1973).

In this chapter, we describe how the thermodynamically open systems that constitute the human organism respond to rapid increases in entropy and activate restorative processes. We discuss how thermodynamics operates in complex biological entities and explain links to Levinas's ethics (Levinas, 2003) to set out a phenomenological basis for the energetic power of suffering.

Understanding phenomena as complex, whereby constituent variables or 'whole-parts' evolve as they interact, necessitates a different way of thinking about causal power, one that recognises causal power as arising from dynamic interactions among constituent parts (Schertzer and Lovejoy, 2011; Rozier and Narteau, 2014). In this framing, causal power is conceived as an emergent property of particular and often myriad, self-organising, dynamic interactions. As biologist Kriti Sharma notes, in a causally complex world 'products depend on processes, processes depend on products, wholes depend on parts, parts depend on wholes, and living beings depend on one another' (Sharma, 2015, p. 1). Entropic overwhelm, experienced as suffering, in this formulation is understood to causally influence the dynamics of internal restorative mechanisms and emergent behaviours, such as seeking help from healthcare practitioners.

The logic of our argument is that in humans as complex biological entities:

• Elevation in entropy can be reversed (it is possible to recover from suffering).
• Elevation in entropy activates internal restorative processes, generated within the biological system, that can reduce entropy/suffering and/or generate recovery.
• Suffering is the felt sense (phenomenological interoception) of elevation in entropy.

- Elevation in entropy can also activate external restorative processes, such as the recruitment of help from other people, to relieve or assist in recovery from elevated entropy/suffering (this does not necessarily equate with cure or recovery from illness, but rather with lowering the level of entropy and felt suffering).
- The experience of suffering can thus be understood as effecting coordination of individual and collective behaviour across healthcare organisations.

While in Chapter 1, we discussed the theoretical and philosophical basis of the explanatory power of conceiving rapid entropic increase as the basis of both suffering and the instigation of restorative processes, here we present a bio-medical account that sets out a theoretical-empiric grounding for a thermodynamic description of system evolution over time. In so doing, we aim to foster epistemic cognitive insights to assist in reconceptualising prior causal modes of thinking about the management and organisation of healthcare. We posit a model that is instead grounded in a clearer understanding of how healthcare processes and practices evolve in entropic flows, that emerge from the interdependencies and reciprocity of bio-medical and organisational dynamics, organising around the attractor of minimisation of entropy production.

Disease and trauma as biological manifestations of elevated entropy

The description of disease and trauma in bio-medicine as equating with elevation in entropy is not new.

Samaras, in 1974, proposed the second law of entropy, whereby organic systems are understood to become more disordered over time, as a global theoretical framework for explaining aging and for identifying the characteristics of human beings 'which can at least retard and possibly stop deterioration of the human organism' (Samaras, 1974, p. 314). He argued that over time the subsystems, organs, tissues, cells and processes that compose the human organism degrade as the body's natural mechanisms for restoring cells does not result in the 'complete restoration and alignment of the cells that make up the body' (Samaras, ibid.), with some imperfections always remaining. Samaras asserted that while these may at first be unnoticeable at a macroscopic level, with time, as more cells are not fully restored, the imperfections accumulate until 'a weak spot occurs in a vital organ and the entire systems collapses' (Samaras, 1974, p. 314). He pointed towards the role of the person's environment, heredity, life style, nutrition and mental state to assist in retarding cellular degradation (entropy development) and thus maximise the health of the subsystems, organs, tissues, cells and processes composing the human organism.

More recently, Schwartz et al. (2020) explain the usefulness of considering pathogenesis in terms of increase in entropy. Understanding the living cell as an entropic material system that releases entropy into its environment, either into the body or into the environment outside of the body, they describe pathologies as when 'entropy cannot be fully exported outside the body and stays inside the body either in the form of intracellular biomass, or extracellular waste produces' (Schwartz et al., 2020, p. 1). They propose that diseases be classified by consideration of the kind of entropy that cannot be excreted, explaining that classified in this way, inflammatory diseases are understood to 'play with entropy through increased heat, biomass synthesis (proliferation of lymphocytes and neutrophils) and secretion of pro-inflammatory proteins (waste products from the cell's point of view)' (ibid., p. 1). They conclude that although cancer and the various degenerative diseases give rise to different symptoms, understood in this way, a remedy against cancer should also be active against degenerative diseases.

Gryder, Nelson and Shepard (2013) focus on entropy as loss of information. They describe the death of an organism as eventuating from biosemiotic entropy, the deterioration of biological sign systems, which they argue, accumulates stochastically over the lifetime of an organism. Describing cancer as 'a disease characterised by the breakdown of cellular systems that exist to maintain, regulate and replicate genetic information' (p. 234), Gryder et al. argue that while cells can be understood from various perspectives, 'the most fundamental genetic system is one of information flow: Communication using signs, codes and signals (biological semiosis, or biosemiosis)' (p. 234). They propose a theory of biosemiosis, 'a working framework for accurately viewing the nature of biological information, its symbolic communication, and the errors which occur in its processing' (p. 234). Gryder et al. suggest this is a useful guide in hypothesis-driven research, arguing that 'casting diseases such as cancer in terms of biosemiotic entropy can aid in interpreting the incoming tsunami of genomic and epigenetic data, in addition to informing the principles that shape future cancer treatment strategies' (ibid., p. 234).

So, a thermodynamic description of disease sits comfortably in the epistemic framing of the medical discourse. We now offer a generalised thermodynamic explanation for how the suffering of disease and trauma can be understood to initiate restorative processes, from within the individual, through to healthcare organisations. Following this, by means of a detailed case study concerned with the response of physicians to a particular intervention in a hospital ED, we demonstrate how understanding reduction in entropy as central to healthcare processes and practice offers practitioners and managers insights into strategies to facilitate improvement.

A thermodynamic explanation of suffering

Broadly stated, a thermodynamic explanation of suffering describes suffering in terms of energy transfers and transformations in the complex (self-organising, dynamic and emergent), biological systems that comprise the human being.

As complex living organisms, humans manifest 'extreme micro complexity' (Morin, 2008, p. 5), in that the cells, molecules, organs and processes of which humans are composed, are also complex 'whole-parts' (wholes and parts of other wholes), that exist through modes of interaction. We characterise these modes of interaction as involving causal powers and mechanisms that dynamically alter the interdependencies of different whole-parts in a structure of relations. In this conceptualisation, the health of humans is characterised in terms of energetic transactions and transformations as each 'whole-part' manages order and disorder. Consequently, human health and the systems or whole-parts constituting the human being can be characterised as thermodynamic phenomena (Melamede, 2008).

In Chapter 1, we described our thesis that suffering in humans can be characterised in thermodynamic terms as a sense-state of elevated entropy production in the body. In this framing, suffering becomes the causal power for activating mechanisms and relations between multiple interacting variables, from the cellular and intrapersonal, to the interpersonal and institutional. These mechanisms minimise or reverse entropy (suffering) by way of introducing intentional, non-random energy that promotes reorganisation and reduces the need for energy consumption. Through these processes, systems can be self-sustained at an orderly distance from equilibrium (Schneider and Sagan, 2005).

Activation of internal and external restorative support for managing increase in entropy is based on: (1) The increase in entropy generating derangement of steady state and loss of *homeostasis* and (2) the person having the capacity to sense this derangement, via the hierarchical integration of signals of entropic elevation, described in bio-medical terms as *interoception*.

Elevation in entropy activates restorative processes via homeostasis

Katzir-Katchalsky provides a useful introduction to the manifestation of entropy in biological systems:

> Life is a constant struggle against the tendency to produce entropy by irreversible processes. The synthesis of large and information-rich

macromolecules, the formation of intricately structured cells, the development of organisation – all these are powerful anti-entropic forces. But since there is no possibility of escaping the entropic doom imposed upon all natural phenomena under the Second Law of thermodynamics, living organisms choose the least evil – they produce entropy at a minimal rate by maintaining a steady-state.

(Katzir-Katchalsky, 1963, p. 43)

Within the human body as a complex biological entity in its 'struggle' against entropy production, entropic increase activates restorative homeostatic mechanisms to maintain functionality at a steady state. This involves three elements: (1) reciprocity, (2) integrated reflexes and (3) information processing. We propose that these three elements respond adaptively to the rate and persistence of entropy production.

Reciprocity and reflexes engage energy flow and force coupling for homeostasis

The initial capacity of the body to respond to sudden increases in entropy is broadly based on two related mechanisms: (1) The flow of energy along gradients, coupled with energetic forces that produce, in their simplest forms, a steady state between two opposing extrema and (2) the action of dissipative structures (thermodynamically open 'whole-parts') capable of reorganising energy dynamics to reverse or slow entropy production by doing work to create order (Mobus and Kalton, 2014).

The first mechanism by which homeostasis is maintained, *reciprocity* of energy around a set-point, is a consequence of the thermodynamic properties of energetic flow and force in non-linear, non-equilibrium (complex) energy systems. Flow and force describe how energy transforms or moves in space and time. Flow is usually along an established potential gradient, for example, the gradient between potential energy and kinetic energy as when an object falls. Force arises from mechanisms such as hydrostatic pressure or electro-mechanical work, as in blood pressure and the work of muscles.

Reciprocity can be illustrated via a brief description of kidney function. A simple model of kidney filtration defines a semi-permeable membrane punctuated with a series of hollow tubes that allow only certain sized molecules to pass from the blood-side to the urine-side of the membrane. On average, over time, the body aims to keep the concentration of different molecules within a 'normal range' in the blood. The filtration by the kidney is affected by the force of hydrostatic pressure created by blood movement, and the concentration difference (flow energy) between molecules in the blood compared to the amount in the urine. Changing the force dynamic can reciprocally affect the flow dynamic and vice versa (Alpern, Moe and Caplan, 2013). The outcome is that despite momentary changes in either force or flow dynamics, on average, the concentration of molecules in the blood remains constant within the normal range for homeostasis via the reciprocal relations of the force and flow mechanisms.

Reflexes, the second mechanism by which homeostasis is maintained, are complicated, multi-system restorative responses, typically described as unconscious or pre-conscious phenomena. Reflexes are an example of dissipative biological elements, like those defined by Prigogine, as structures where reciprocal force and flow dynamics act irreversibly on energy metabolism to convert energy into work. This work creates information-rich products that increase the organisation of the system and lowers system entropy (Prigogine, 1980).

Consider a person who has tripped over. The sudden change in energy flow from potential energy to kinetic energy, sensed in mechanical and vestibular organs, signals loss of balance. The change in flow gradients activates electrochemical forces in the form of neuro-muscular action potentials from the spinal cord that generate work, in the form of muscle contractions to regain and maintain balance. Sometimes this response may be so swift that we only register the slightest sensation of balance being perturbed. The ability to restore balance involves many layers of sensing and response, where reciprocal flow and force couplings are integrated to generate wide ranging responses across the organism, that convert energy in muscle cells to the work of contractions, to restore the steady state of balance.

Many homeostatic responses are the result of even higher integrated modes of sensing and reacting that, for the most part, involve the central nervous system of the body. For these responses, layers of adaptive reorganisation are required across many systems of the body to maintain and restore steady state. In these instances, simpler 'cause and effect' inputs and outputs are insufficient for management of increased entropy. Instead, an informed response is required that takes account of multiple streams of inputs and simultaneously assesses the consequence of different responses across integrated systems. This necessitates information processing.

Integrated dissipative structures of homeostasis involve new levels of information processing and interoception

As hierarchical integration of reflexive and dissipative mechanisms increases, the interaction of 'whole-parts' becomes more complicated. This is because, as England (2013) notes, survival is contingent on an organism having sophisticated integrative capabilities that can assess 'whole' and 'part' consequences of shifting homeostatic dynamics, to ensure energy consumption is at its lowest effective level, thus minimising entropy. Such integrative processes rely on the third mechanism by which homeostasis is maintained: *Information processing*. Information about the environment, availability of energy for work, and the overall minimisation of entropy production must be processed and integrated. In complex organisms, the primary seat of information processing is in the central nervous system: The brain.

Information theory (Shannon, 1948) and physiology inform understanding of how the central nervous system is able to quickly process tremendous amounts of information. Researchers (Zimmermann, 1989) note that the central nervous system and brain compress enormous amounts of bits of information (data). One important consequence of these information processing capabilities is that rules which filter out or eliminate predictable information (e.g., information that confirms a system is operating within homeostatic boundaries), can enable more readily, identification of surprising or unexpected information.

Within the unexpected or surprising information, there is a higher probability of finding useful information about a changing state of the system. In biological systems, it is more efficient (less energy demanding) to monitor and link restorative actions to breaches of the extrema of homeostatic ranges, than to monitor all individual changes, moment-to-moment, which are of no biological consequence. Thus, in a complex living system, where lots of data require continuous monitoring and adjustment, some of the most useful information about the state of the system will be found in data signalling *disorder*.

In bodily systems, much biological monitoring is performed unconsciously. There is no need for higher level system responses if the monitors are sensing that the systems are operating within homeostatic boundaries. We become 'aware' or conscious of bodily-psychological processes most often when homeostatic boundaries are persistently or dramatically transgressed – a phenomenological process described in bio-medical terms as *interoception*. It appears that our cognitive awareness is triggered by interoceptive states that essentially register 'surprising' biological states. This is when there is a high probability that the information being conveyed in the breach is 'useful' because it is, on the background of the other predictable measures, a 'surprise' to the monitoring structures. In addition, hierarchical integrated monitoring processes are signalling that lower-order dissipative and reflexive mechanisms to maintain homeostasis have been overwhelmed and thus the circumstances may require a whole of organism response to avoid continuing entropic decay.

Information integration in the central nervous system

Higher order synthetic and adaptive information processing, balance efficiency, accuracy and the amount of work being done in the organism to reduce overall long-term average entropy production.

At higher orders of integration, simply responding to fluctuations around extrema will not necessarily achieve an optimal outcome. Without a major coordinating force within the central nervous system, competing drives from multiple simultaneous derangements may be found to result in faulty, uncoordinated and ultimately disastrous responses by the organism to its predicament. Simply stated, without the informational integration achieved by the central nervous system, an entity as complex as a human being, would cease to function, or at least function inefficiently in terms of entropy production.

Neuroscientist Karl Friston (2010) has developed a theory, called the 'Free Energy Principle' that offers a plausible explanation of how biological organisms minimise entropy production in higher order information processing. According to his Free Energy Principle, biological organisms can minimise entropy production by reducing the gulf between their expectations and sensory inputs. Friston suggests that minimising the 'surprise' aspect of information management in the higher order integration of an organism's myriad complex processes provides a survival advantage in the face of inevitable entropic decay.

Friston posits that the Free Energy Principle assists the biological entity to maintain a steady state of homeostatic boundaries, by minimising the amount of surprise encountered both within its internal makeup and in relationship to its environment, and that this minimises entropy production (which he terms 'free-energy metabolism'). To achieve this, the agent (to use Friston's nomenclature) has control over two key things: (1) They can change sensory input by manipulating their environment to change the stimulus affecting the sensory field (a 'bottom-up' approach) or (2) they can change their perception of what is causing a particular sensation by changing their internal schema of causation (a 'top-down' approach).

Friston's work describes how the hierarchically integrated layers of neuronal organisation use sensory data to continually optimise an internal model of the world by way of probabilistic inference. The inferred conceptual question continually being interrogated is: How well does this model actively predict the world, based on the evidence arising from the information arriving from the senses? By optimising either the 'bottom-up' or the 'top-down' information, harmonisation of the interiority and exteriority of experience results in a reduction in informational entropy and surprise.

The importance of feeling states

Interoception is not simply a 'data synthesis and analysis' of entropy consequences of our 'cause and effect' perceptions of our environment or the signalling from internal homeostatic derangement.

We tend to describe surprising entropic states, not in terms of physical or physiological processes, but instead with a range of words that describe a 'feeling'. We are more likely to say, 'Ow, that hurts' in response to a burn, than to describe the underlying physical phenomena providing the sensation for the burn.

The feeling state conveys that the sudden entropic increase has been a significant enough surprise to have signalled, within the hierarchical information processing of our brain and central nervous system, that an assault to our bodily functions may require our conscious attention to coordinate a whole-of-organism response to ameliorate or avoid it. Interoception of bodily senses is coordinated in brain areas including the limbic, insula and anterior cingulate structures of the brain (Kleckner et al., 2017). These centres are critical to homeostasis and also generate the primary emotional responses including 'fright, flight, fight', coordination of sleep and dreaming, memory and social cognition (Rajmohan and Mohanda, 2007). There is an emerging understanding that interoceptive pathways activate restorative physiological responses to restore homeostasis and modulate social cognition (Hubler, 2014).

Critical to our thesis, Pinna and Edwards (2020) systematically reviewed studies on interoception and emotional regulation to find that they are deeply integrated, with emotional responses modulating how interoceptive and high-order state-representations select for different behavioural choices.

One way the emotions may shape behavioural responses is through dynamic interference within hierarchical integrative structures. Pakhomov and Sudin (2013) suggest that emotions provide a powerful initiation of essential chaotic dynamics within our neural hierarchies, to allow for decision-points to form, from which choices can be made. By extension, this means the sensations underlying suffering, such as pain, mechanical stress, muscle fatigue or disability, by the process of interoception, are inculcated with emotive sensations, to which we ascribe a feeling. Our response to a given insult may require choices between competing demands. To make a choice, we require conditions that allow for a change of mind or an over-ride of prior decision pathways. Emotions may create an important part of the necessary hierarchical conditions within which choices are made possible.

Summary of the thermodynamic explanation of suffering

In this section we explored in some detail a bio-medical explanation of how entropy effects the structure of complex biological entities and the interdependencies and information processing that make meaning of the dynamic evolution of these structures through time. As Morin (2008) has described, the 'extreme micro complexity' of the whole-parts that constitute the living structures of humans, exist through modes of interaction which, as shown in the preceding exploration, include (but are not limited to) reciprocity around set-points, reflexes, and information processing that are organised to maintain a steady state of homeostasis. The bio-medical research we have outlined establishes a theoretical-empiric foundation from which to elaborate the proposition that suffering, the felt-sense phenomenon of homeostatic derangement due to excessive entropy production, is a causal power that can reorganise system responses to a loss of homeostasis.

Human health, in this framing, is characterised in terms of entropic transactions and transformations responding to an interplay of order and disorder within homeostatic boundaries. Research into biological systems suggests that internal homeostatic mechanisms over time can degrade or become overwhelmed such that disease and illness manifest. Our proposition is, that at the point of overwhelm there are whole-of-organism integrative structures that can coordinate a 'call for help' to seek out restorative interventions from the surrounding environment, to try to arrest or slow entropy production and so restore homeostasis.

In support of this proposition, we explored the role of interoception as a possible mechanism to activate biological, physiological, psychological and social systems of relations in response to 'surprising' derangements of steady states of homeostasis. Interoceptive outputs have causal powers to activate mechanisms and relations between multiple interacting variables from the cellular and intrapersonal to the interpersonal and institutional. Some research suggests that the common goal for any of the myriad ways in which these variables might evolve over time is likely geared towards selecting states of being that are least-entropic and thus confer a longer-term survival advantage.

The turn outward for help, when internal restorative processes and mechanisms are insufficient to meliorate entropy production, necessarily activates systems of social interaction in an environment that is prepared to provide interventions in support of the relief of suffering. In this turn, the suffering of the individual becomes an entropic flow, expelled and reverberating, through the structures of healthcare which are organised in response to the call for help – the patient–practitioner relationship, the ED, the hospital and so on.

At these scales of organisation (the ED, the hospital and so on), how people make sense of the causative elements of suffering, and the interventions that will resolve excessive entropy production (thus, relieving suffering), become contingent on the qualities of higher order organisational mechanisms for managing entropy between people in the healthcare context. How and why social structures of healthcare exist and can successfully intervene in response to the call of suffering are explored in the following sections.

How suffering (elevation in entropy) can elicit help from others

Where humans encounter an overwhelming or continuous and dangerous increase in entropy perturbing a steady state of homeostasis, and where internal homeostatic responses have failed to restore or reverse the entropic increase, the whole organism must be coordinated to make sense of, and respond to, this ongoing threat.

There would be little need for the variety of healthcare institutions if the total potential for recovery from suffering was contingent upon internal bodily energetic mechanisms. Instead, there are myriad insults, injuries and aberrations of the living substance, that without the cooperation and input of external energies and agencies would hasten disintegration, or at the very least result in continued suffering, and humans, for the most part, appear driven to avoid suffering.

The theoretical-empiric bio-medical explanation of how thermodynamics function in complex open systems, set out in previous sections, informs complexity thinking about how structures of relations responding to entropy and homeostasis might organise, from within individuals to across collectives of human activity, and provides a basis for theorising the modes of interaction and evolutions of those systems across scale. Understanding individuals and healthcare organisations as complex entropic entities that are organised around the attractor of seeking to reduce elevated entropy, means that to make sense of how we manage entropy in patients, we must also be mindful of the consequences of entropy production for healthcare practitioners and organisational dynamics, into which the entropy of suffering from patients is expelled.

We have proposed that humans have hierarchies of systems that monitor and respond to changes in steady state via homeostasis, and that the nervous system coordinates whole of organism responses to sudden changes in entropy production that signal harm (or potential harm), in which the common expression is suffering. As a function of this sophisticated hierarchical coordination, emotions and feelings are critical to directing people who are suffering, to seek assistance, under the foreknowledge that non-random energies can be introjected into disorganising systems to halt or reverse entropy. Thus, a secondary agency may be sought in the form of a healthcare practitioner, to assist in reducing the elevated entropy in the person who is suffering.

In the hospital ED, where extreme states of rising entropy are concentrated, staff bear witness to many powerful expressions of suffering. The events taking place in an ED show that there are almost limitless conditions assailing the human organism that may generate suffering. Derangements of physical organisation (cuts, broken bones, blocked blood vessels), physiological (hormone imbalances, septic shock) and biochemical processes or mental processes, constitute examples of the many ways by which the complex human organism may express catastrophic disturbances of function that exhaust or overwhelm homeostasis. No matter the origin, what is in common, is that all those suffering manifest excess entropy production, with this macro-state 'calling' to the external environment for assistance (energetic intervention).

Levinas's ethics: A phenomenological basis for the energetic power of suffering

The call for assistance when one's biological systems are unable to reduce elevation in entropy necessarily requires other people who are willing to assist. While thermodynamically we might refer to the power of energetic interventions to assist in restoring biological functions, this does not explain the willingness of others to help, nor necessarily the investment by human civilisations in the structures of healthcare.

In understanding responses to suffering as a human relational phenomenon, we turn to Levinas's conception of how human beings relate to one another through an ethics of responsibility.

In both a thermodynamic and ethical sense, the groan, can be thought to elicit a response from the other to offer immediate relief, not for the sake of extending life, but primarily, to alleviate suffering. In Levinas's ethical philosophy, one is ethically bound to seek to resolve suffering in the other, which elicits from ourselves the foreknowledge of the uselessness of our own suffering and the drive to extinguish it.

Interestingly, support for understanding humans as motivated to help someone who is suffering can be found in research that explores the psychology of human suffering, in disciplines such as neuroscience and evolutionary psychology. Researchers in these disciplines propose human compassion evolved as an emotional response to the perceived suffering of others, and that compassion is grounded in our biology, and vital to the health of individuals and the survival of our species (Goetz, Keltner and Simon-Thomas, 2010). In their comprehensive review, Goetz, Keltner and Simon-Thomas suggest the major evolutionary arguments for the evolution of compassion 'converge on the hypothesis that compassion evolved as a distinct affective experience whose primary function is to facilitate cooperation and protection of the weak and those who suffer' (ibid., p. 351). Their definition of compassion as 'the feeling state that arises in witnessing another's suffering and that motivates a subsequent desire to help' (ibid., p. 351), closely aligns with Levinas's ethics of responsibility. However, the direction of this body of research into compassion differs from our work, in that the focus is less on the power of suffering to activate a response and more on understanding factors relating to compassionate responses.

Bringing together Levinas's insight and a biological thermodynamic perspective, the organising principle of the response to the suffering of self and others might thus be characterised as iterative interdependencies tending toward an economy of energetic expenditure in which entropy is slowed or reversed.

Healthcare, as socially organised systems of response to suffering, wherein people with expert knowledge and a desire to relieve suffering are grouped together (general practitioner clinics, dentists, physiotherapists, hospitals, EDs and so on), constitutes an efficient emergent mechanism by which to promote recovery. This reflects the same energetic principles of efficiency and minimisation of entropy that we have described in the biological processes within people. Indeed, Wallace (2009) has described how thermodynamics and entropic flow can explain evolutions of complex social structures over time. Hence, entropy appears as a central attractor within many complex phenomena at different scales, around which thermodynamic structures of relations can be described.

The entropic and ethical dimensions of the clinical consultation

In our framing, the clinical consultation between the healthcare practitioner and the person seeking care, has its antecedence in the causal power of suffering. According to Levinas's ethics of relationship, and a thermodynamic, bio-medical understanding, interaction between the patient and practitioner represents the fulcrum of the structure of relations called into being by the suffering of the person seeking healthcare.

The clinical encounter is where interaction between the patient and healthcare practitioner takes place. It is 'the point at which decisions about diagnosis and treatment are made, and during which caring takes place' (Dieppe, Rafferty and Kitson, 2002, p. 279).

Described in terms of energetic transactions and transformations, the clinical consultation represents a self-organising, dynamic and emergent encounter between complex entropic entities. The patient, or person seeking care, is conceptualised from a thermodynamic perspective, as a complex biological being who is experiencing elevated entropy and is thus suffering (or who is seeking to manage or avoid future suffering). The 'care' they seek, in thermodynamic terms, is a reduction or reversal in elevation of entropy, that can be achieved by activating necessary energetic transfers. The healthcare practitioner is not only able to help, they have the necessary expertise to offer non-random energetic interventions, but motivated to help through their stance within the Levinasian ethical knot of responsibility.

Healthcare, entropy and fractality

New models implicate new ways of seeing and doing. The value of viewing healthcare in a new way lies with the potential for gaining beneficial insights that lead to improvement in practice. One of the advantages of our ComEntEth theoretical framing of healthcare is, that by explaining complex interactions and emergence in terms of entropic transactions and transformations, we offer a unified way of perceiving trauma and illness, alleviating treatments, and the multitude of complex relationships and their causal interdependencies, implicated in healthcare. While complexity perspectives have influenced, in myriad ways, understanding of both bio-medicine (e.g. Seely and Christou, 2000; Seely, Newman and Herry, 2014; Tuffin, 2016) and healthcare organisational dynamics (e.g., Plsek and Greenhalgh, 2001; Sturmberg, 2019; World Health Organization, 2006), our model is the first, to our knowledge, to conjoin bio-medicine and organisational dynamics around management of elevated entropy (suffering), as the central attractor guiding healthcare processes and practices.

Understanding interactions in healthcare (such as between patient and practitioner), as energetic exchanges, constitutes an integral perspective that encompasses biological, social and psychological aspects of healthcare. Entropy in our framing, serves as a communicative 'common denominator', as it enables us to conceptualise suffering (illness and trauma) and healthcare related interventions, no matter the nature of the assault/derangement, nor the area of specialisation of the healthcare practitioner, in terms of entropic exchanges. This can assist practitioners from various specialised knowledge disciplines to work together more effectively.

Furthermore, understanding reduction in suffering/entropy as facilitated by sourcing energy from surrounding environments (such as that constituted by healthcare practitioners in a healthcare setting), highlights the importance of effective management of entropy levels between healthcare practitioners. This means, rather than view bio-medical care of the patient as separate from the dynamics associated with management of healthcare organisations (organisational culture, behaviour, learning and development), both bio-medicine and workplace dynamics, are perceived as together implicated in healthcare provision.

Our ComEntEth model reveals how healthcare provision arises through interdependencies and reciprocities between bio-medicine and organisational dynamics. It emphasises the importance of the quality of connections between stakeholders (patients, practitioners, managers, policy designers) and shows how daily interactions lead to habitual attitudes and collective behaviours or norms of processes and practices. The quality of daily interactions is shown to impact all involved and to significantly influence the capacity of healthcare practitioners to reduce suffering/entropy in the suffering patient.

The complexity concept of fractality (Mandelbrot, 1977) provides a way of highlighting at different levels of focus, reciprocality between biology, patient care and broader stakeholder interactions. We observe fractality in the way the open thermodynamic system under review, such as a cell or person, self-organises and dynamically interacts with its surrounding environment, drawing energy from this surrounding environment, as it manages entropic levels.

At the first fractal level, the system within the biology of the individual (such as a cell or organ) dynamically interacts with the internal surrounding biology to source energy and manage entropy. At the second fractal level, the whole person (suffering patient) dynamically interacts with their environment, including healthcare practitioners, to source energy and manage entropy. At the third fractal level, the healthcare clinic, practice or department dynamically interacts with the broader healthcare environment (hospital, national healthcare fora and so on) to source energy and manage entropy. At the fourth fractal level, the hospital or national healthcare fora dynamically interacts with the prevailing socio-economic-political environment to source energy and manage entropy.

The principle common across all four fractal levels is that management of entropy is achieved by entropic exchanges with the surrounding system/environment. In thermodynamic terms, for this to occur effectively, the system under review requires its environment to have the capacity to provide the energy necessary to minimise entropic increase.

Our model indicates how entropic increase can potentially flow across multiple entities/surrounding environments, as energy is drawn from a succession of 'whole-parts' and their surrounding environments. The model emphasises how management of entropy has contingent and interdependent evolving effects.

For overall healthcare performance to be effective, healthcare organisations need to consider the entropic impact of habitual processes and practices of getting things done. Recognising that the capacity of practitioners to reduce patient entropy is impacted by organisational dynamics and broad policy and economic functions, attention to the influence of management practices on management of entropy across the whole organisation is essential.

Case study: Introduction of the 4-Hour Rule/National Emergency Access Target

Having set out the philosophical and bio-medical basis and logic of our ComEntEth conceptualisation of healthcare, we now turn from theoretical exposition to practical illustration. We do this by means of a case study.

This case study comprises three parts: Background; narrative presentation of a scenario; and interpretive commentary. The narrative presentation is based on verbatim accounts of physicians, of their experiences of the impact of a time-based administrative intervention, the 4-Hour Rule/ National Emergency Access Target (4HR/NEAT) on ED processes and practices in Australian public hospitals.

Our intention in presenting this case study is to demonstrate in an accessible manner how our ComEntEth model can be used to (1) critically analyse practice, (2) identify mechanisms by which processes and practices arise and (3) identify strategies that facilitate the capacity of those involved to more successfully manage entropy levels in the provision of healthcare.

Background to the introduction of the 4HR/NEAT in Australia

In the early 2000s, overcrowding and access blockages were identified by a range of governments and national colleges of medicine, as the most serious issues faced by EDs in the developed world, because of a negative effect on the timeliness and quality of patient care (Derlet, Richards and Kravitz, 2001; Forero, 2008; The Royal College of Emergency Medicine, 2018). In the United Kingdom, the National Health Service (NHS) addressed this problem by introducing a target that 'no-one should be waiting more than four hours in accident and emergency from arrival to admission, transfer or discharge' (The NHS Plan, 2000).

In 2008, a delegation of clinicians from Western Australian (WA) hospitals examined the critical factors in the success of the NHS in utilising a 4-Hour Target to address overcrowding and access block in UK EDs. The delegation concluded that the 4-Hour Target was a useful reform that could be implemented and adapted to the Australian context. Following this, in 2011, the Australian Commonwealth Government implemented a National

Emergency Access Target (NEAT), colloquially known as the 4-Hour Rule (4HR) (Council of Australian Governments, 2011).

The 4HR/NEAT mandates that ED processes for 85% of ED patient presentations should be completed within four hours. The 4HR/NEAT constitutes a performance measure and meeting the target has been tied to the Australian Commonwealth distribution of funds for health.

The reform generated widespread strong negative emotional responses from physicians, and this led to one of us (Le Plastrier, 2019), undertaking research into why the reform caused so much angst. Over 18 months, Le Plastrier conducted a series of one-to-one, face-to-face, semi-structured interviews to gain the views of ED physicians about how the 4HR/NEAT impacted on ED processes and practices, and specifically, on their experience of (1) the clinical encounter, patient interaction and safety, (2) collegial interactions and workplace dynamics, and (3) ED productivity.

Despite representing a range of different levels of experience and disciplines across medicine, the physicians presented homogeneous experiences of the effect of the rule on the clinical encounter. Each privileged the patient–physician relationship above other dynamics and demands of the ED environment and held a powerful sense of responsibility for the wellbeing and lives of each patient. They described the environment of the ED and the dynamics of relationship between physicians and other ED staff as having changed significantly with the 4HR/NEAT. There was unanimous agreement that the impact of the 4HR/NEAT at the level of the individual clinical encounter had the potential for adverse effects on both physician and patient.

The physicians expressed negative views about the impact of the 4HR/ NEAT on the clinical encounter, patient interaction and safety and collegial interactions and workplace dynamics. They spoke of the emotional toll of being forced to make what they felt were unsafe clinical decisions, pressure from colleagues to prevent patients 'breaching' the 4HR/NEAT, and of how when they become stressed by these competing demands, they retreat into clinical work at the expense of broader situational awareness across the department. The physicians' narratives suggest they hold in tension a range of pragmatic issues, such as identification of the particularities of each patient's case and maintaining patient safety, against external drivers to meet the time-based target of the 4HR/NEAT and managing the consequences of high demands on their intellectual and emotional resources.

What follows is a composite, indicative narrative (Kuhn, 2018) that summarises the physicians' views by bringing their responses together as one voice.

Indicative narrative: Perceptions of ED physicians on the impact of the 4HR/NEAT on the ED

In the ED clinical encounter, I introduce myself, and the patient and I size each other up and work out how we'll communicate. That's a deliberate step for me. It sets the scene for the consult. As information is gained I make decisions about what direction to take the consultation and the diagnostic tests to be ordered. The 4HR/NEAT makes this process stressful because I undertake it with a sense of a time limit.

So, I'm assessing caseness, looking at the evolving symptoms and severity. I'm engaged in a continuous process of clinical assessment and reassessment and wondering if the medications I've prescribed are worth it and if I've missed something. I'm feeling pressured to make decisions quickly and being questioned by the nurses about what I'm doing.

With the focus of managers on key performance indicators and compliance with the 4HR/NEAT, there's pressure to get things done before I've had time to really think about what's needed and a relentless flow of people to see and I mightn't have had any dinner.

In terms of productivity, I appreciate that it's important to ensure patients are seen in a timely way and resources used appropriately, so that we minimise any poor outcomes in terms of morbidity and mortality. I just can't ascitic tap, pleural drain or lumbar puncture patients without constant awareness of using resources. But, if this place gets busy the triage nurse starts ordering bloods off everyone, ordering everything on the panel. When the triage nurse has ordered everything, that sets up more work. For example, if troponin comes back positive even when it wasn't indicated in the first place, we have to do something about it – talk to cardiology and run a stress test.

Care of the individual patient is the driving force. If I'm not getting that right, in the midst of all that I'm doing, I feel compromised. The irony is that as the department gets more congested, getting people out does help, so the 4HR/NEAT is good in that way. But if I get patients out to somewhere without them being fully worked up then I wouldn't feel they are safe, so I'd worry about them anyway and not actually reduce my cognitive load. We don't always find out what's wrong with them immediately, but our job is to make sure that when they leave here, they are safe. I worry that faster processing and assessment could lead to errors in diagnosis.

We have all these people here in ED, trying to get patients out in 4-hours and it feels like this causes more pressure and no-one stands back to look at what else is going on. There's increased stress in ED staff, degraded relationships between staff, such as between doctors and nurses, greater administrative burden, more reliance on junior doctors and increased bullying around 4HR/NEAT compliance.

Some things can be solved quite quickly and other things take time. I had a patient, a young person, first presentation to psychiatric services, who came into ED. We talked for at least an hour, and I said 'That's lots of information, I'd like to go and talk to someone who knows you'. I wanted to speak with the consultant. Then the nurse manager asked me what was happening with the patient, and I said, 'I don't know yet, we still haven't talked to family, we have no background, and I'm hopeful that we can get this person home to avoid them being admitted – but we need more time'. I'm pretty senior as a registrar, nevertheless, the nurse manager instructed me to 'make the decision now'. I felt under huge pressure to make a disposition decision and the logic wasn't related to patient welfare at all. So, there's a lot of bullying going on around 4HR/NEAT compliance.

I think clinical performance is much broader than the patient–physician relationship. It includes how well we assess someone, interact with colleagues, use good evidence-based patient management, give appropriate referrals and do this with awareness of resourcing limitations. So, for example, if one of my registrars sees a patient and calls a gastroenterologist, and then the gastroenterologist bites their head off for calling them, that's not OK. I think people forget that. Working under the 4HR/NEAT often leads to conflicting, rather than collegial ways of interacting. But, if you're in charge of the ED, it's hard to maintain situational awareness when it gets really busy,

The idea that you are meant to process so many patients within 4-hours means high stress levels. Patients come in, get triaged and see the ED doc. They might have bloods taken and require specialist input. This all takes time. There are things outside of my control. I can't determine how quickly the pathology or imaging comes back. Often, it's the results of these tests that determine what needs to be done. Things like fluids take a bit of time. I don't think 4-hours is an unreasonable time expectation in terms of the patients as they don't want to spend all day in the emergency department if they don't have to. Unit management staff add to the stress and the pressure and make me feel like I'm not doing a good job when they say 'You need to hurry up'. I can't necessarily hurry my patient interaction and the time it takes to have tests done and the results come in, or to answer patient questions and reassure them.

Interpretive commentary

This indicative narrative references a number of entropic states and exchanges, relating to those involved in the ED (such as that of the patient, physician, nurse and nurse manager). Analysing the various entropic states and exchanges (entropic flow) allows detailed insights into the social interactions and emergent collective behaviours that constitute the ED. In addition, the narrative provides evidence of the 'micro-state' entropic processes affecting the performance and behaviour of individual people within the ED and how these might feed into, 'bottom-up', the overall entropic 'macro-state' performance of an ED or hospital.

The sense of feeling pressured and stressed by the imposition of the 4HR/NEAT is pervasive in this narrative. This indicates raised levels of entropy in the physician. From the initial meeting with the patient, to decisions about diagnostic tests, caseness and disposition, all are described as impacted by a need to be mindful of time constraints. Feeling stressed lowers the morale of the physicians and may have an impact on their interoception, thus raising their entropy levels. Worry about correctness of decisions made under pressure leads to higher cognitive and emotional loads and this too increases entropic levels. Higher levels of stress/entropy were perceived to reduce the capacity for situational awareness as the physicians focus more intensely on their clinical work. Feeling stressed and pressured tended to translate into degraded and conflictual exchanges with staff, which may degrade communicative exchanges, further exacerbating entropy production in the physicians and across ED staff with whom they interact.

Though the indicative narrative expresses the physicians' views, we can infer from their narrative that people in different positions in the ED view the 4HR/NEAT differently and that different factors may cause increased entropy in the different actors. For example, the narrative suggests that managers might be feeling stressed due to difficulties in getting the physicians to work in such a way that the ED can comply with the 4HR/NEAT. Similarly, it might be that the triage nurse feels stressed and 'orders bloods off everyone' in an attempt to facilitate faster passage of patients through the ED. However, as these tests offer little additional useful information about the disease/trauma of the patient they increase informational entropy in the department.

Thermodynamically, an effective clinical encounter is characterised by a meaningful exchange of information, leading to effective determination of caseness and generation of appropriate actions to bring relief of suffering (reduction in entropic increase) in the patient, with maximal dissipation and minimal rise in overall ED and hospital entropy.

In contradistinction, the physicians' view in this narrative is that the 4HR/NEAT engenders a thermodynamically ineffective clinical encounter. They consider the 4HR/NEAT constricts the capacity of the physicians to engage in meaningful exchange of information, identify caseness and generate appropriate actions to reduce the suffering of the patient, contributing to a rise in entropy across the ED. From the perspective of viewing suffering as characterised by increase in entropy, we can appreciate staff across the ED are also suffering, as they seek to attend to patients and comply with the 4HR/NEAT.

The pervasiveness of raised entropic states of the various actors generates overall entropic increase across the ED. In a reciprocal manner, this then further increases the entropic load of the physicians as they engage with patients and reduces overall ED productivity by impairing their ability to diagnose and appropriately manage their patients.

With implementation of the 4HR/NEAT geared to address ED over-crowding and access block, this reform evidences a desire by those who developed and introduced it, to reduce elevated entropy/suffering in patients by improving access to the entropy reducing influence of medical profes-sionals. Lessening of ED congestion, and facilitation of access to hospital care means that more patients are better positioned to be given quality care (energetic interventions designed to reduce elevated entropy) in a timely manner.

Although motivated by a shared impetus, reduction in patient suffering/elevated entropy, the reform is judged by the ED physicians as having a nega-tive influence on the capacity of healthcare to facilitate care of patients. From the perspective of our ComEntEth conceptualisation, reduction in entropy is facilitated through energetic interventions provided by the healthcare practitioner, and for this to be done effectively, the practitioner and broader healthcare context ought to be functioning with the least amount of entropy production. So, although those involved in developing and implementing the 4HR/NEAT and the ED physicians share the aim of optimal care for patients, in the physicians' view, unforeseen consequences of the 4HR/NEAT across healthcare mitigate against effective strategies to reduce suffering/elevated entropy. A complexity perspective warns against expectations that interven-tions into complex phenomenon will have a linear relationship between intervention and outcome, and to expect surprising effects, which in this case, is rise in entropy of the physicians and the ED, and thus less capacity to effectively lower the entropy of the patients.

Recourse to consideration of phase space/phrase space reminds us that as all those who are impacted by this administrative reform make sense of it according to their own schemas and discuss their views with colleagues, over time certain habits of thought and taken for granted assumptions become accepted as 'how things are' and 'how things ought to be'. These then shape how the various stakeholders engage with and judge, the effectiveness of the 4HR/NEAT. In the physician's narrative, we see a contrast between the phrase space of the physicians and that of the nurses and nurse managers. With the physicians describing how they feel pressured in attempting to fulfil their duties under the requirements of the 4HR/NEAT, it appears their phrase space supports viewing the 4HR/NEAT as an administrative time-based intervention that has a negative impact on the care of patients. As depicted by the physicians, it appears the nurse and nurse manager's phase space has more emphasis on the need to comply with this time-based intervention. This might be because they would face disciplinary action from their line managers if the 4HR/NEAT requirements are not met.

An advantage of a phrase space analysis is that it does not privilege or demonise one interpretation, but lays out the range of individual interpretive responses, so that they become available as 'knowable objects', amenable to further reflection and analysis. In this way, making a phrase space analysis available to the participants concerned with the situation (here, the physicians, nurses, nurse managers and administrators of the ED), facilitates mutual reconceptualisation, where all those involved might be invited to contribute to developing a new understanding and appreciation of the situation.

Importantly, having participants engage in a non-judgemental way in developing new understandings can facilitate improved connections between those involved. In this way, phrase space reconceptualisation can facilitate communicative connectedness, and conversely, improved communicative connectedness engenders an increased commonality of phrase space, across the different actor groups. With both improved communicative connectedness and increased commonality of phrase space, entropy levels of all involved are minimised.

In the physicians' narrative, we see evidence of how the ED arises through the nature and quality of communicative exchange between multiple stakeholders. In the ED, as in other human endeavours, relationships with other people really matter and these are dependent on the nature and quality of communication between all who are involved. The narrative indicates how, via communicative connectedness, sophisticated forms of joint action, such as diagnosis and treatment of patients are engendered.

The physician's narrative calls attention to a range of conversational exchanges and depicts how the nature and quality of these shape attitudes and how things get done in the ED. The beginning of the narrative describes awareness of the importance of the introductory conversation with the patient in setting the initial conditions for the patient–physician relationship. This demonstrates implicit understanding of the importance of communicative connectedness. In terms of the imposition of the 4HR/NEAT, the narrative depicts a sense of disconnect between the physician and nurses/nurse managers, with the physician referring to nurses/nurse managers as attempting to limit their capacity to undertake their professional responsibilities. The expressed sense of a degradation of relationships between the various professional healthcare groups, such as between physicians, nurses, nurse managers and administrators, indicates potential negative influences on social interactions and thus on the day to day activities as well as on the future unfolding of the ED. Lack of coordination between staff, for example, could lead to an increase in the number of patient complaints and increased risk of medical errors. There could also be an increase in workplace dissatisfaction, with an increase in resignations and higher staff turnover, and the requirement for greater funds to be given over to staff recruitment and onboarding (orientation and socialisation).

Communicative connectedness can be conceived as a conscious, adaptive response to felt uncertainty, as people participate in dynamic, unfolding complex processes. It shares hierarchical organisational principles with the integrative meaning making functions of the human brain.

In organisations such as a hospital and ED, there are stylised forms of fostering communicative connectedness. Formally these activities might include meetings and review processes, while informally, communicative connectedness is reinforced via casual conversational opportunities, such as at the nurses' station. From a communicative connectedness perspective, strategies to reduce the physicians' stress, as well as that of all the ED staff, would include increased formalised processes to develop a stronger consensually agreed strategy around 4HR/NEAT compliance. Importantly, these formalised processes would need to allow scope for the self-organising responsive strategies of the individuals involved, to effect reductions in entropy.

Interestingly, research conducted in Australia in which successful implementation of the 4HR/NEAT was achieved in terms of its proposed endpoints of reduced wait times and improved quality of care, highlight that success was borne of factors such as staff enthusiasm and engagement, staffing levels and clinical and administrative leadership (Silk, 2016). Factors such as these, are indicative of the communicative connectedness necessary for people within organisations, to build consensual strategies that change practices and self-eco-organise new ways of doing things together to achieve positive clinical outcomes.

Conceptualising the impact of the 4HR/NEAT in terms of entropic flow shows that viewed from the physicians' perspective, the 4HR/NEAT has the potential for negative psychosocial and financial consequences. Thinking in terms of entropic flow draws attention to how micro-events, such as one-to-one interactions between physicians and nurse managers, can evolve into macro trends, such as medico-legal cases, loss of staff, and associated increase in financial burden.

Significantly, in addition to illustrating how awareness of entropic states can foster insights into social interactions and emergent collective behaviours, this interpretive commentary illustrates how cognisance of phrase space and communicative connectedness directs attention towards ways by which raised entropic levels might be mitigated, such as via strategies that foster non-judgemental interactions and common understandings.

References

Alpern, R. J., Moe, O. W. and Caplan, M. (Eds) (2013) *Seldin and Giebisch's the Kidney*. Amsterdam: Elsevier Academic Press.

Council of Australian Governments (2011) *The National Health Reform Agreement: National Partnership on Improving Public Hospital Services*. www.federalfinancialrelations.gov.au/content/npa/health_reform/national-agreement.pdf

Derlet, R., Richards, J. and Kravitz, R. (Feb. 2001) 'Frequent Overcrowding in US Emergency Departments'. *Academy of Emergency Medicine*. 8(2):151–155.

Dieppe, P., Rafferty, A. and Kitson, A. (2002) 'The Clinical Encounter: The Focal Point of Patient-Centred Care'. *Health Expectations*. 5(4):279–281.

England, J. (2013) 'Statistical Physics of Self-replication'. *Journal of Chemical Physics*. 139:121923.

Forero, R. (2008) 'Block and Overcrowding: A Literature Review Prepared for the Australasian College for Emergency Medicine (ACEM)'. Australasian College for Emergency Medicine.

Friston, K. (2010) 'The Free Energy Principle: A Unified Brain Theory?'. *Nature Reviews*. 11:126–137.

Goetz, J. L., Keltner, D. and Simon-Thomas, E. (2010) 'Compassion: An Evolutionary Analysis and Empirical Review'. *Psychological Bulletin*. 136(3):351–374.

Gryder, B. E., Nelson, C. W. and Shepard, S. S. (2013) 'Biosemiotic Entropy of the Genome: Mutations, Mutations and Epigenetic Imbalances Resulting in Cancer'. *Entropy*. 15(1):234–261.

Hubler, A. (2014) 'Interoceptive Sensibility Predicts the Ability to Infer Others' Emotional States'. *PLOS One*.

Katzir-Katchalsky, A. (1963) 'Nonequilibrium Thermodynamics'. *International Science and Technology:*43–49.

Kleckner, I. R., Zhang, J., Touroutoglou, A., Chanes, L., Xia, C., Simmons, W. K., Quigley, K. S., Dickerson, B. C. and Varrett, L. F. (2017) 'Evidence for a Large-Scale Brain System Supporting Allostasis and Interoception in Humans'. *Nature: Human Behaviour*. 1:69.

Kuhn, L. (2018) 'Complexity Informed Social Research: From Complexity Concepts to Creative Applications'. Mitleton-Kelly, E., Paraskevas, A. and Day, C. (Eds) *Handbook of Research Methods in Complexity Science*. Cheltenham: Edward Elgar Publishing.

Le Plastrier, K. (2019) 'The Entropy of Suffering: An Inquiry Into the Consequences of the 4-Hour Rule for the Patient–Doctor Relationship in Australian Public Hospitals'. Doctoral thesis, Western Sydney University.

Levinas, E. (2003) 'Useless Suffering'. Bernasconi, R. and Wood, D. (Eds) *The Provocation of Lévinas: Rethinking the Othe*r (R. Cohen, Trans). London: Routledge.

Mandelbrot, B. (1977) *The Fractal Geometry of Nature*. New York: Freeman.

Melamede, R. (2008) 'Dissipative Structures and the Origins of Life'. Minai, A. and Bar-Yam, Y. (Eds) *Unifying Themes in Complex Systems IV*. Berlin: Springer.

Mobus, G. and Kalton, M. (2014) *Principles of Systems Science*. New York: Springer.

Morin, E. (2008) *On Complexity* (R. Postel and M. Kelly, Trans). New Jersey: Hampton Press.

Pakhomov, A. and Sudin, N. (2013) 'Thermodynamic View on Decision-Making Process: Emotions as a Potential Power Vector of Realization of the Choice'. *Cognitive Neurodynamics*. 7(6):449–463.

Pinna, T. and Edwards, D. J. (2020) 'A Systematic Review of Associations Between Interoception, Vagal Tone and Emotional Regulation: Potential Applications for Mental Health, Wellbeing, Psychological Flexibility and Chronic Conditions'. *Front Psychology*. 5(11):1782.

Plsek, P. E. and Greenhalgh, T. (2001) 'Complexity Science: The Challenge of Complexity in Health Care'. *British Medical Journal*. 323:625–628.

Prigogine, I. (1980) *From Being to Becoming: Time and Complexity in the Physical Sciences*. San Francisco: Freeman.

Prigogine, I. and Lefever, R. (1973) 'Theory of Dissipative Structures'. Hagan, H. (Ed) *Synergetics*. Fachmedien Wiesbaden: Springer.

Rajmohan, V. and Mohandas, E. (2007) 'The Limbic System'. *Indian Journal of Psychiatry*. 49(2):132–139.

Rozier, O. and Narteau, C. (2014) 'A Real-Space Cellular Automation Laboratory'. *Earth Surf. Processes Landforms*. 39(1):98–109.

Samaras, T.T. (1974) 'The Law of Entropy and the Aging Process'. *Human Development*. 17:314–320.

Schertzer, D. and Lovejoy, S. (2011) 'Multifractals, Generalized Scale Invariance and Complexity in Geophysics'. *International Journal of Bifurcation Chaos*. 21(12).

Schneider, E. and Sagan, D. (2005) *Into the Cool: Energy Flow, Thermodynamics, and Life*. Chicago: Uni Chicago Press.

Schwartz, L., Devin, A., Bouillaud, F. and Henry, M. (2020) 'Entropy as the Driving Force of Pathogenesis: AS Attempt of Diseases Classification Based on the Laws of Physics'. *Substantia*. 4(2).

Seely, A., Newman, K. and Herry, C. (2014) 'Fractal Structure and Entropy Production Within the Central Nervous System'. *Entropy*. 16(8):4497–4520.

Seely, A. J. E. and Christou, N.V. (2000) 'Multiple Organ Disfunction Syndrome: Exploring the Paradigm of Complex Nonlinear Systems.' *Critical Care Medicine* 28:2646–2648.

Shannon, C. E. (1948) 'A Mathematical Theory of Communication'. *Bell System Technology Journal*. 27(3):379–423.

Sharma, K. (2015) *Interdependence*. New York: Fordham University Press.

Silk, K. (2016) *The National Access Emergency Target: Aiming for the Target But What About the Goal?* Canberra: Deeble Institute Issues Brief.

Sturmberg, J. (Ed) (2019) *Embracing Complexity in Health: The Transformation of Science, Practice, and Policy*. New York: Springer.

The Royal College of Emergency Medicine (2018) *Emergency Medicine Briefing: Making the Case for the Four-Hour Standard*. The Royal College of Emergency Medicine. The NHS Plan (2000) Cm 4818–1.

Tuffin, R. (2016) 'Implications of Complexity Theory for Clinical Practice and Healthcare Organisation.' *British Journal of Anaesthesia: Education.* 16(10): 349–352.

Wallace, T. (2009) *Wealth, Energy and Human Values: The Dynamics of Decaying Civilizations from Ancient Greece to America.* Bloomington: Author House. Pp. 469–489.

World Health Organization (2006) 'To Err Is Human'. *Patient Safety.* DOC:1.4.

Zimmermann, M. (1989) 'The Nervous System in the Context of Information Theory'. Schmidt, R. F. and Thews, G. (Eds) *Human Physiology.* Heidelberg: Springer.

3 Improving Entropic Flow in Healthcare Organisations

Introduction

Our beginning point, in thinking about how entropy production can be minimised in healthcare organisations, is the day-to-day experiences of all those who are involved. Our understanding of daily experiences as fundamental to organisational manifestation and evolution echoes that of Melucci:

> Daily experiences are only fragments in the life of an individual . . . yet almost everything that is important for social life unfolds within this minute web of times, spaces, gestures and relations.
>
> (Melucci, 1996, p. 1)

We concur with Melucci (1996), in understanding that it is via daily interactions – experiences and behaviours – that habitual attitudes and collective behaviours, or norms of healthcare processes and practices are created. As organisational theorist Ralph Stacey puts it:

> We must work to clearly understand just what it is that we are doing together in our groups, or in our organisations, that leads to the emergent patterns that are our experience. The patterns of behaviours are the organisations. They happen as a result of all the things that people are thinking and feeling and doing.
>
> (Stacey, 2002/2003, p. 28)

Healthcare work has long been recognised as stressful. Just as the suffering of illness or trauma is correlated with increase in entropy, so too, is increase in stress correlated with increase in entropy. In this chapter, our focus is on how the practice of healthcare can be improved by minimising entropy development across the individual humans whose experiences and behaviours create healthcare organisations.

DOI: 10.4324/9781003197454-3

The work related sense of stress and concomitant elevated entropic levels of those who make up healthcare organisations, provide insights into how people in the various organisational groups are working together in the provision of healthcare. Analysing the entropic states and exchanges in, and between, the people who constitute healthcare organisations, provides a way of gaining insights into the social interactions and emergent collective behaviours by which healthcare arises. From this analysis, we can also learn about principles and strategies for minimising entropic development in healthcare organisations and the individual humans who create them.

In this chapter, we interpret organisational dynamics in terms of entropic exchanges. We explore the role of entropy in shaping how things get done in the daily life of healthcare organisations. To better understand how to effectively manage the complexity implicit in the provision of healthcare, we interrogate energetic transactions and transformations (entropic flow) in a non-mathematical, metaphorical manner. With reference to major themes in healthcare and organisation studies literature, we identify principles and practices for minimising entropy production across stakeholders.

ComEntEth model revisited

A brief recapitulation of our ComEntEth (Complex Entropic Ethical) theoretical framing of healthcare is useful at this point, to set the scene for showing how comprehension of organisational dynamics as entropic exchanges can lead to beneficial insights into strategies for improving the provision of healthcare.

In Chapters 1 and 2, we explained how viewed from the perspective of our ComEntEth model, whatever the scale of focus, global system, sector, organisation, department or the individuals involved, healthcare complexity arises through myriad entropic transactions and transformations that cohere around efforts to reduce suffering or entropic levels in patients. Furthermore, we outlined how focus on entropy engenders an integral perspective that encompasses biological, social and psychological aspects of healthcare, and links the provision of bio-medicine with organisational dynamics.

In our model, healthcare organisations and the individuals involved, are recognised as exhibiting key features of complex phenomena: They have their own purposes; consist of networks of interacting agents; interact with and within environments; choose what they take notice of; act in accord with their own schemas of rules; discover the responses that their actions evoke, and use this information to revise their schemas and behaviour (Stacey, Griffin and Shaw, 2000). As complex entropic entities, healthcare organisations and the individual humans by which they are constituted, are conceptualised as engaging in a continual dialogue with their environments (including other individuals, departments, institutions, sectors), while at the same time dynamically self-organising in response to changing circumstances, and endeavouring to keep their internal entropy at manageable levels.

In Chapter 2, we presented a bio-medical explanation of the role of entropy in human interoception, illness, trauma and suffering. We explained how a person experiencing disease and trauma is a complex living entity whose internal entropy has exceeded manageable levels, and who requires energetic interventions to assist in reducing entropy levels so as to mini-mise the threat to life. In showing how reduction in entropy is facilitated by sourcing energy from surrounding environments, and specifically, the role of the healthcare practitioner in this process, when internal homeostatic responses are insufficient or overwhelmed, we indicated the importance of effective minimisation of entropy levels between healthcare practitioners and others involved in creating healthcare organisations, in order to sus-tain the potential of the practitioner and organisation to reduce the entropy (hence, suffering) of the patients they serve.

The conditions in which a suffering person reaches outwardly to another for care were described in terms of Levinas's self-other responsibility. In concurring with his philosophy of an ethical *a priori* relational imperative, we view this as operating through the interdependencies and interactions of the people seeking and providing healthcare, and, by extension, founda-tional to the healthcare imperative.

As explained in Chapter 1, consideration of the processes and practices of healthcare, as ethically contingent energetic transactions and transforma-tions or entropic flow, provides a way of identifying the dynamic capacity, character of interactions and longevity of healthcare organisations, be they departments, clinics, sectors and so on. If each functional unit of healthcare is viewed as an ethical and entropic entity, we can have expectations with regard to its past, present and future. We can examine how the energetic input into the entity meet, or fail to meet, the energetic requirements of the entity. Where the energetic requirements are not met, we can expect to find evidence of raised entropy in the organisational unit and ineffective practices that ultimately endanger patient health, rather than ameliorate suf-fering and enact the ethical knot of self-other responsibility.

In this framing, awareness of entropic reverberations across the practice of healthcare is important as it allows us to gain information about the adap-tive 'self-eco-organising' of the people and organisations involved, as well as indications of how to better manage entropic flow.

Healthcare organisations and the individuals involved, require and rely on, energetic inputs to support the processes of self-organisation. Energy is expended through the activities necessary to maintain organisation (minimi-sation of entropy) and support regeneration. Paradoxically, these activities also generate entropy. As organisations and individuals undertake processes of self-organisation while in dialogue with their environments (they are self-eco-organising), entropic reverberations can be expected across the multiple interactions via which healthcare emerges.

Our argument, therefore, is that minimising energetic expenditure, and thus entropy levels, across these multiple interactions, supports effective management of the entropy levels of the practitioner, and this places them in the best position to deal with the patient's elevated entropy.

In order to minimise entropy levels across healthcare organisations, however, we need to consider both the patterns of interactions through which the organisation emerges and the daily experiences of those involved. From a complexity perspective, daily interactions not only shape future emergence but they are set within iterations of interaction. As Geoffrey Vickers, in studying complex patterns of social organisation, puts it 'the standards by which human order is defined are in part culturally set by the societies which they organise' (Vickers, 1984, p. xx). Vickers draws attention to the way that the standards of self-expectation and mutual expectation that more or less govern social interactions (ideas about how healthcare practitioners should act), at any one time, can be viewed as emergent from histories of patterns of interaction. These patterns, as sociologist Norbert Elias (1978) proposes, emerge out of an interweaving of people's intentions and plans (Stacey, 2002/2003). It is interesting that, though both Vickers' and Elias' work predates the emergence of the complexity sciences, they share a conception of human society as self-organising, dynamic and emergent.

Though daily interactions and experiences, and patterns of interaction are understood as reciprocal, we separate them out for ease of examination. In beginning the chapter with a focus on the daily experiences of stress in healthcare practitioners, we first demonstrate how bio-medically stress is evidenced as increase in entropy within human beings. We then discuss identified workplace stressors for people working in healthcare.

We next discuss some widely recognised characteristics of organised patterns of interaction within healthcare organisations, and suggest how these might play with increasing or decreasing stress/entropy levels across healthcare organisations.

Building on this basis, we explore how sources of increased stress can be identified in healthcare organisations, by interrogating entropic flow across the multiple relationships involved in the processes of organising in healthcare in terms of four interpretations of entropy: Energy unavailable for useful work, uncertainty, disorder/dispersal and loss of information.

Via analysis of two vignettes, we demonstrate how conceptualising healthcare in terms of our ComEntEth model, focuses attention on entropic flow and in so doing, can stimulate new insights that can lead to improvement in practice.

Entropy and stress in everyday life

It is commonplace for people to talk about feeling stressed or under tension from relational demands, pressures to get things done, personal goals and expectations and so on. We do not hear people say 'My entropy levels are elevated', 'I'm having difficulty managing my entropy' or 'My boss continually transfers their excess entropy to me'. Similarly, when ill or suffering, and in need of medical intervention, we do not say 'My entropy levels are exceeding my biophysical capacity and I need urgent medical energetic intervention'. In scientific and medical research, in the same way that suffering is linked with rapid significant elevation in entropy, stress and entropy are recognised as linked. Just as biological/psychological disintegration signals significantly elevated entropy, so too, does stress indicate pressure on everyday dynamic self-organisation and increase in entropy. In this sense, stress can be described as physical, mental or emotional tension in response to demanding circumstances.

Given that the word 'stress' is commonly used in daily life to describe phenomena identified as increased entropy in scientific and medical research, and given the creative metaphoric propositional style of our argument, we begin by presenting indicative bio-medical research that confirms a correlation between stress and entropy.

Peters, McEwen and Friston's (2017) research into why stress causes diseases, draws on recent developments in theoretical neurobiology. Defining stress as uncertainty, and uncertainty, as entropy, they present an information-theoretic account of stress. In sum, they argue that reducing uncertainty (entropy) requires cerebral energy. Greater cerebral energy demands extra energy from the body. If the sense of uncertainty remains unresolved, Peters et al. conclude that 'a persistent cerebral energy crisis may develop, burdening the individual by "allostatic load" that contributes to systemic and brain malfunction (impaired memory, atherogenesis, diabetes and subsequent cardio and cerebrovascular events)' (p. 2). Through detailed biomedical exposition, their research demonstrates links between prolonged stress, understood as a prolonged sense of uncertainty or raised entropy, and the potential development of disease.

Focusing on research into emotional responses, Pakhomov and Sudin (2013) demonstrate mathematically and conceptually, how emotional responses are linked with changes in energy flow that effect the activity of cells and organs. Their evidence shows that emotional and higher cognitive functions can operate as 'top-down' controllers of the responses of reflex systems in our bodies that attempt to drive our physical systems back towards usual states. As a consequence, our memories, thoughts, and intentions, arising from mind and consciousness, have access directly to physical systems in our bodies that can provide the work for re-establishing appropriate levels of entropy. Pakhomov and Sudin also show how, from the other direction, derangement of physical systems measured as an entropic function of stress, can be understood to directly impact, bottom-up, our state of mind and also be used to drive our physical being towards least dissipative states and more equanimous emotional states.

Blons et al. (2019) conducted research into psychophysiological responses to stressors. Their findings indicate a relationship between cognitive load and stress, with neurophysiological complexity altered by mild stress, reflected in change in entropy of the cardiac output signal.

Bienertova-Vasku et al. (2016) developed Stress Entropic Load (SEL) as an approach to stress measurement, that is based on 'thermodynamic modelling of entropy production, both in the tissues/organs and in regulatory feedbacks' (p. 1). Drawing on entropy as their departure point, the authors argue that their holistic thermodynamic model of health and disease makes it possible to calculate stress, by quantifying 'its accumulation based on the cumulative production of entropy associated with a given stressor or a combination of stressors in a specific individual' (p. 11).

The previous examples of bio-medical research all conclude that experience of increased stress correlates with elevated or increased entropy. Their work is indicative of a substantial body of research that supports our assertion that stressors put pressure on the dynamic self-organisation of the individuals and collectives involved in healthcare, and so raise entropy levels and contribute to less energy available for useful work, greater uncertainty about what to do, increased disorder and loss of information. It is important to note too, that although extensive medical research exists about the role of sustained stress and raised entropy in the development of illness, that research is beyond the scope of this book.

Consideration of stress in terms of entropic flow means that rather than stress being viewed as a function of an individual's ability to cope, or as a problem attributable to singular cause and effect mechanisms between sets of deterministic interacting variables, we are drawn to consider the mechanisms through which entropy manifests in the whole (organisation, department, institution, sector). This approach offers an integrative perspective, where one could metaphorically trace or map the movement of stress (raised entropy) across a whole organisation (department, sector) and identify leverage points to most effectively improve whole of organisation functionality.

Stress/increased entropy in healthcare practitioners

We have argued that entropic reverberations across healthcare organisations can serve to minimise or magnify entropy, as experience of stress, in healthcare practitioners. Increased entropy (stress) is understood to negatively affect the capacity of practitioners to provide high quality health care. In this section, we present indicative research showing that stress (increased entropy) in practitioners is well known as a phenomenon of concern, and further, that there is substantial evidence demonstrating that increased stress (entropy) in practitioners has a negative effect on healthcare performance. Drawing on recent studies, we discuss identified workplace practitioner stressors and explain how these act as entropic magnifiers.

Stress in healthcare practitioners has long been an issue of concern. Stress related to one's workplace or profession is well recognised and the healthcare professions are identified as among the most stressful of occupations (Riley et al., 2018). Riley et al. note that compared with the general population, physicians in the United Kingdom experience high levels of stress and burnout. A recent study of US physicians noted 46% exhibited at least one symptom of burnout, while a Canadian study found 80% of physicians suffered moderate to severe emotional exhaustion (Kumar, 2016). Studies across the range of healthcare professions similarly identify high levels of stress in practitioners. For example: Podiatry (Tinley, 2015), physiotherapy (Lindsay et al., 2008) and speech pathology (Fimian, Lieberman and Fastenau (1991).

Stress, however, cannot be simply conceived in terms of profession or workplace conditions. Typically, stressors are characterised as relating to internal (personality traits of individuals) or external (situation or processes external to the individual) factors (Australian Medical Association (AMA), 2011). Susceptibility to stress, and to particular stressors, is known to vary between individuals. Studies have identified how the personal qualities that underpin the professional success of medical practitioners (such as dedication, commitment, responsibility, altruism) can become a source of pressure and increase the risk of doctors experiencing stress problems (AMA, 2011; WMA, 2015).

Nevertheless, it is the stressful work situations that have been identified as the most significant risk factor for healthcare practitioners' mental and emotional health (Koinis, Giannou and Maria, 2015).

As healthcare practitioners take care of people's lives, mistakes can be catastrophic and irreversible. Practitioners are expected to bring a calm and focused state of mind to their care of patients (in other words, minimal entropy). However, this is not always the case because practitioners are not only susceptible to the same stressors as the general population, but also prone to additional stress related to the peculiarities of their professional responsibilities (Familoni, 2008). As stated in 'Stress Management for Nurses' (Brunero et al., 2006), in their daily work, nurses 'confront emotional and professional demands that are unimaginable to the wider community . . . spending your working life taking responsibility for the quality of people's lives and their deaths is a heavy burden' (p. 4). Similarly, the Australian Medical Association's 'Position Statement on Health and Well-being in Doctors and Medical Students' (AMA, 2011) notes how encounters with patients and their families can be a potent source of stress when doctors are involved in 'dealing with suffering and death, in emotionally charged clinical situations'.

These 'confrontations' to emotional and professional demands within the patient–clinician relationship harbour an ethical dimension to the stressors experienced by healthcare workers and augur the risk of moral injury (Griffin et al., 2019). Researchers have found that practitioners experience moral stress in every day practice stemming from inter-professional trust and opportunities to listen to patients and their carers (Bartholdson et al., 2016) that can affect perception about the quality of care and the effectiveness of decision-making in professional teams (Atabay, Cangarli and Penbek, 2015). Ulrich, Taylor and Penbek (2013) argue that there is a lack of emphasis on the moral hazards of clinical practice and that, for nurses, this increases levels of stress and may affect nursing staff retention. Importantly, in Griffin et al.'s review of literature on moral stressors and moral injury, organisational and institutional factors were reported by people experiencing adverse effects of moral injury, including out-of-touch leadership, difficulty identifying threats in the environment, dehumanisation of others, and loss of trust in external relationships including partners, communities, and governments.

Recent studies identify significant stressors beyond those implicit in direct care of patients. Escalating bureaucratic requirements and administrative duties, workforce shortages, reduction in resources, increasingly litigious environments, rapid advances in medical knowledge and challenges to expertise by patients and other healthcare providers are widely reported by physicians as important causes of stress (Kumar, 2016; Riley et al., 2018; World Medical Association (WMA), 2015). These stressors, in comprising threats to practitioner autonomy, professional identity and access to resources, contribute to increasing entropic load in healthcare practitioners, and so negatively impact practitioners' capacity to hold patient entropy and offer effective entropy reducing interventions in patients.

There is substantial evidence that stress, in having deleterious effects on practitioners, negatively affects the quality of care of patients and the confidence of the general public in healthcare providers. The British Medical

Association's publication 'Work related stress among senior doctors – review of research' (2000) concluded that a significant proportion of doctors experienced significant stress and that this was inimical to the doctors' health and to their care of patients. Koinis et al. report that the negative effects on the mental–emotional health of healthcare practitioners can be attributed not only to their work environment but also to the coping strategies they employ (such as quitting). Other studies note that when intense stressors exceed tolerance thresholds, there is risk of reduction in quality of care (Berland, Natvig and Gundersen, 2008; Dewa et al., 2017).

The link between health practitioner stress and quality of patient care is perhaps best expressed by West and Coia (2019), in their review of the factors that impact the wellbeing of medical students and doctors, 'Caring for Doctors, Caring for Patients'. They conclude that 'The wellbeing of doctors is vital because there is abundant evidence that workplace stress in healthcare organisations affects quality of care of patients as well as the doctors' own health' (p. 12). The multiplicity of studies into the effects of stress on a range of different healthcare practitioner professionals suggests this insight might be expanded to 'The wellbeing of *healthcare practitioners* is vital because there is abundant evidence that workplace stress in healthcare organisations affects quality of care of patients as well as the practitioners' own health'.

Importance of minimising stress/entropy across all healthcare practitioners

In response to the prevalence of high levels of stress, healthcare practitioners are exhorted to maintain well-being and to optimise all factors that affect their biological, psychological and social health. Documents produced by national and global bodies in response to the prevalence of significant stress in healthcare practitioners, typically focus on strategies that individuals might take to promote their resilience, such as seek medical or counselling treatment, or resilience or healthy life style training (AMA, 2011; BMA, 2000; WMA, 2015).

Such approaches to management of stress, implicitly regard practitioner stress as a function of the individual practitioner's ability to cope, or as a problem attributable to singular cause-and-effect mechanisms. In contrast, the approach we take in this book is to consider the mechanisms through which entropy arises across the whole organisation. In this framing, practitioner stress can be viewed as symptomatic of increased entropy across the sector, organisation or department.

Some studies into stress in healthcare practitioners, however, do recognise the interlinked, cumulative and systemic nature of work place stressors.

These studies advocate attending to strategies, beyond those directed at the individual practitioner, to improve practice culture and workplace conditions. Indicative strategies include modifying organisational structure and work processes (reasonable working hours, promotion of interdisciplinary team work and communication skills) and addressing cultural dynamics (power, politics and bullying within the practice) (Kumar, 2016). Riley et al. conclude that it is imperative that organisations promote 'compassionate and supportive work cultures . . . in addressing the dynamic interplay between the personal, professional and organisational sources of stress and distress in GP's' (p. 6).

We expand this strategy to argue that addressing the dynamic interplay between the personal, professional and organisational sources of stress and distress in all who are involved in healthcare is necessary to reduce individual stress and minimise entropic flow across healthcare organisations. A complexity perspective, in noting that relationships between constituent parts give rise to collective behaviour and phenomena, directs our attention to a broader consideration of how stressors arise and might be addressed in healthcare organisations. A complexity understanding of healthcare focuses our attention on how cultural dynamics and workplace norms arise through local interactions between individual actors. Individuals and their contexts (clinics, departments and so on) in this framing, are understood to emerge out of modes of relating. Relational exchanges between people, constitute energetic transactions and transformations, which taken over time and across organisations, give rise to entropic flow, through which emergence manifests.

From a complexity perspective, strategies that assist in minimising entropy or stress and managing the challenges of practice, such as maintenance of well-being, biological, psychological and social health, should be advocated as important for all involved in healthcare, not just healthcare practitioners. Interestingly, the Rochester Campus of the Mayo Clinic took this perspective in introducing 'serious leisure' to patients, physicians and the medical workforce generally (Dieser, Edginton and Ziemer, 2017).

Dieser, Edginton and Ziemer explored how leisure opportunities within the daily experiences of patients and healthcare practitioners lowered patient stress and relieved practitioner burnout. Taking a serious leisure approach, however, means a particular approach to engaging in leisure activities. According to sociologist Robert Stebbins (1982), who proposed a theoretical framework for classifying and explaining different types of leisure (serious, casual and project-based), serious leisure is based on commitment to developing special skills, knowledge and experience. This approach to leisure highlights the importance of a deep emotional and cognitive commitment by the participant in the leisure activity, to the stress-relieving effects of engaging in the leisure activity.

When a healthcare practitioner's stress or entropy is minimal, their capacity to hold and transform a patient's elevated entropy (suffering), by offering timely and pertinent interventions, is maximised. Minimal entropy in practitioners, facilitates, what physicians describe as, 'pattern recognition', where they are able to immediately recognise the correct diagnosis, based on an automatic, non-analytic integrative process. Pattern recognition can be understood as commensurate with intuition, 'gut feeling' and insight, in that pattern recognition encompasses non-conscious cognitive processing, in drawing on pre-existing knowledge and experience and comes about without intentional effort (Hogarth, 2010). Intuition can be viewed as a means of reducing cognitive load (and hence entropic level) because it allows practitioners to respond instantly with confidence in their knowing.

Optimal clinical decision making has been described as an interplay between overtly drawing on logical information processing and intuitive knowing (Nalliah, 2016). As pattern recognition or intuition relies on past experience, this can at times lead to bias, so practitioners need to quickly and easily bring together logical information processing and intuitive knowledge. Increased entropy, through being tired, overwhelmed or excessively busy, impedes logical thinking and privileges intuition, and so negatively affects clinical decision making (Rongjun, 2016).

Recognised characteristics of patterns of interaction within healthcare organisations

Fundamentally, organisations constitute collectives of human activity, where the patterns of interaction are shaped by the actors involved, along with historical, social and cultural contexts and assumptions. Scholars across a range of disciplines (psychology, sociology, social sciences, philosophy, anthropology, human geography, complexity sciences) contribute to the study of the patterns of interaction, or processes and practices, through which organisations arise. Much analysis has engaged with questions about the agency of the individuals involved and how agency plays with organisation structure, or established rules, processes and norms. Sociologist Anthony Giddens argues that both agency and structure reciprocally shape patterns of interaction:

> Human consciousness is conditioned in a dialectical interplay between subject and object, in which man [sic] actively shapes the world [organisation] he [sic] lives in at the same time as it shapes him [sic].
>
> (Giddens, 1971, p. 21)

Giddens draws attention to how what people do in an organisation is conditioned by the prevailing rules, processes and norms, and how reciprocally, the prevailing rules, processes and norms are brought into being and reproduced by the actions and behaviours of the individual agents.

Study of organisations remains a contested discourse concerning 'features of organisations [that] will be noticed or ignored, emphasized or discounted, seen as important, or dismissed as irrelevant' (Grey, 2005, p. 123). Assuming that 'how we see the world, determines how we act in it', we can understand theory (how we see the world) as critically important in shaping strategies of action (practice), that condition experience in an organisation.

In broad terms, the range of perspectives brought to the study of organisations, implicate views on structure and agency. Sociologist Max Weber (1947), in reacting against brute indiscriminate forms of authority over employees (power, coercion and fear), advocated rational-legal authority where compliance is secured through codified rules, procedures and duties. Bureaucratic structures based on rational-legal, formal and hierarchical authority, carry a sense of humans as rational beings.

If, in considering organisations as collectives of human activity, we include human rationality and sense making capabilities in the concept of 'human activity', we can understand organisations as existing through the distributed sense making capabilities of all involved. This perspective highlights the importance of strategies that foster conversational exchanges and communicative connectedness and thereby utilise the sense making of those involved.

A raft of approaches to management of people in organisations have evolved over the past 50 or so years, that value the cognitive, creative, ethical and responsive capabilities of human agents. This valuing of agency is demonstrated in theories that view organisational processes and practices in terms of communicative relational exchanges between people as self-determining, rational, self-conscious and socially conscious human beings. Here, who talks to whom, and who trusts whom, are recognised as shaping how things get done in an organisation. Sociologist Etienne Wenger (1998), for example, proposed that things get done in an organisation via 'communities of practice' where people in an organisation (department, clinic), regularly interact as they seek to improve their shared practice.

Similarly, Hirotaka Takeuchi and Ikujiro Nonaka (2004) proposed a theory of organisational knowledge creation as a way to promote organisational learning. In their theory of how organisations process knowledge and create new knowledge, Takeuchi and Nonaka recognise the importance of humans as creators of knowledge, via a process of interacting and sharing ideas:

'communities of interaction' contribute to the amplification and development of new knowledge. While these communities might span
departmental or indeed organisational boundaries, the point to note is
that they define a further dimension to organisational knowledge creation, which is associated with the extent of social interaction between
individuals that share and develop knowledge creation.

(Takeuchi and Nonaka, 2004, p. 166)

Takeuchi and Nonaka conceive knowledge creation in an organisation as
occurring through a 'spiral' involving individuals and their contexts and
they develop a model that explains how individual 'tacit' knowledge is
converted into explicit knowledge, able to be codified and used by the
wider organisational community. It is this conversion process that Nonaka views as necessary to organisational knowledge creation. Organisational learning or knowledge creation is important because it constitutes
the means by which an organisation enhances its resilience, adaptability,
employee job satisfaction and productivity and efficiency (Clegg, Kornberger and Pitsis, 2005).

Takeuchi and Nonaka's main interest is in learning how best to support
practical strategies (including critical review of organisation structure) to
foster organisational learning or knowledge creation. Organisation structures that support human agency, from the perspective of organisational
learning and development, are those that facilitate communicative interaction and whole person engagement.

In recent years networking by individual agents, whereby individuals
choose whom they will source for information and who they will share information with, have been identified as significant in supporting how things get
done in an organisation. That individuals are able to engage in networking
evidences agency, and concomitantly, individual agency is enhanced through
networking.

Whole person engagement by organisations necessitates an organisational response to, and management of, ethical experiences of the people
from which the organisation emerges. Silva et al. (2008) advocate for the
role of clinical ethicists in healthcare organisations to assist with managing pressing organisational issues related to resource allocation, staff moral
distress, conflicts of interest, and clinical issues. Enhancing organisation
ethics is, in the view of Nelson et al. (2010), synergistic with the quality
improvement aims of many healthcare organisations.

This range of theories about the processes and practices of getting
things done in organisations highlights how even in bureaucratic organisations, where formal authority is embedded in hierarchies of oversight and

responsibility (CEO, section head, department head, medical director, clinical director), communicative connectedness conditions structure, and thus individual agency.

Healthcare organisations embody characteristics of bureaucratic, hierarchically structured organisations, that also function through relational exchanges between rational, creative and knowledgeable individuals. Codified rules, procedures and duties can serve to contain entropy production in those working in healthcare organisations, by providing secure parameters of guidance about what and how things should be done. Communicative connectedness, enabled via various forms of social exchange, can also support containment of entropy production, by providing further information and facilitating the means of getting things done. So, in this reading, both bureaucratic functions and social relations serve to manage entropy production by managing uncertainty.

However, beyond this in-principle observation, we recognise that the means by which entropy production in healthcare practitioners might be quelled or exacerbated are infinitely subtle and complex. A number of issues inevitably arise as rational, creative and knowledgeable people interact in organisations. Notably, as all involved attempt to assert their individual sense of identity, have their views and interpretations of events accepted by others, and gain access to resources, there is contestation about what, and how, things should be done, even in healthcare with its focus on assisting suffering patients. Power relations are thereby inevitable in the daily life of healthcare organisations. Power, attached to formal roles within bureaucratic hierarchical arrangements, exerts a compelling influence, such as via codification of rules, procedures and duties, and managing access to resources. Power is also enacted through the actions of individuals expressing their sense of agency (such as commitment to assist the suffering patient). Thus, bureaucratic (formal) and socially interacting (informal) modes of organisation shape the patterns of interaction within healthcare organisations.

Entropic indicators in healthcare organisations

In this section, we introduce 'entropic indicators' as a useful way to identify mechanisms that exacerbate or minimise entropy development, together with strategies for minimising entropic flow across healthcare organisations.

Taken together, study of entropy in physics, chemistry, biological thermodynamics, neurobiology, cybernetics and information theory, suggests that in current formulations, 'entropy' is discussed and interpreted in four principle ways, as unavailable energy, uncertainty, disorder/dispersal and information loss. While these interpretations overlap, they can be conceptually distinguished from each other, and we find this useful in our theorising of the role of entropy in healthcare organisations. We treat these four interpretations metaphorically, as 'entropic indicators' that provide evidence of how entropy is expressed in organisations, and we draw on them to analyse entropic flow and generate insights into how to improve management of complexity in healthcare.

The first entropic indicator, *unavailable energy*, refers to when energy is not available, due to being used in ways that do not support the overall needs of an entity. This might highlight, for example, processes and practices where individuals are so busy hiding their limitations or maintaining their reputations, that much of their energy is not available to contribute effectively to the activities that best support the practice of healthcare.

The second entropic indicator, *uncertainty*, refers to how certain or uncertain a person is about how things might turn out, and therefore, what steps they might take next. Although uncertainty is to be expected, living entities, in learning from past experiences, carry expectations about future activities. When situations evolve that are a long way removed from what was expected, or when alternative future events appear equally likely or probable, people experience a heightened sense of uncertainty. Energy becomes unavailable because it is put into seeking further information, re-evaluating and re-organising. As an entropic indicator, higher levels of *uncertainty* might be seen in a situation where the circumstances or environment are surprisingly different from what was expected, or where there are significant unknown elements at play. For example, if a certain medicinal intervention causes an unexpected detrimental reaction, or if the current government funding policy might be about to change.

The third entropic indicator, *disorder* or *dispersal*, describes entropy changes in terms of energy dispersal across an entity. As noted in Chapter 1, Rudolf Clausius one of the founders of the study of thermodynamics, proposed that thermodynamic processes can be understood as an alteration in the arrangement of the constituent parts of an entity or system and that the internal work associated with these alterations can be quantified energetically by a measure of entropic change (Clausius, 1867).

With it being the nature of all complex entities to tend over time to disorder, energy must be expended on systems and processes to sustain the operational capacities of units, departments, organisations and sectors. Just as we described in Chapter 2 with respect to the bio-medical processes and systems that maintain homeostasis, organisations need to attend to those activities and ways of relating that support their operation within preferred operating boundaries. This is necessary energetic consumption that serves to maintain more orderly systems, expels entropy production to the environment successfully, and supports the continuing adaptive require-ments of employees and the organisation to respond to the demands and changing environments inherent in the provision of healthcare.

We also find interpreting *disorder* as *dispersal* is useful for identifying situations in healthcare organisations where energy must be employed in attending to arrangement of the parts (institutions, departments, clinic, sec-tors), beyond that to be expected in maintaining order in complex entities, with their tendency to become disordered over time. An example of energy being employed in unnecessarily attending to disorder/dispersal is where energy might be put into attending to a micro-state of one component of a healthcare organisation, to the detriment of the collective efforts of the whole organisation to relieve the suffering of the patient. Or where, with high turn-over of senior staff, there are repeated re-structures of the organ-isation. The effects of these additional energy requirements might be that critical tasks are not undertaken in a timely manner, some activities need to be repeated or that critical organisational or patient information is lost.

The final entropic indicator, *information loss*, refers to completeness and fidelity in communication of information or data. As introduced in Chapter 1, entropy as *information loss*, proposed by Claude Shannon (1948), relates to information generated by the source, but not received. In our metaphorical interpretation, *information loss* might occur, for exam-ple, when incomplete communication about diagnosis and treatment of a patient causes unnecessary harm, or when data storage and communica-tions systems so encode, compress and transmit data that critical details about patient history are lost.

Alternatively, too much data presented without the necessary hierarchi-cal and integrative information processing capabilities, creates 'data with-out knowledge'. Ultimately, data are only useful if they express something meaningful about the underlying processes from which they are gener-ated. Without systems and processes in place to 'make sense' of streams of healthcare data, information loss occurs. An example of this is the patient record details collected during admission. Streams of nursing, allied health, medical, vital statistics, and demographic information are collected, often at the time of admission, that would take time to digest. The overwhelming data load means that important information may be difficult to discern from less relevant data, and so important information is lost.

Analysing entropic flow in the practice of healthcare

Through theoretically informed critical reflection on two vignettes, we demonstrate how entropic indicators can identify factors that contribute to increase in stress/entropy and offer propositions for nudging the practice of healthcare towards more optimal outcomes.

We explore circumstances and mechanisms whereby unavailable energy, uncertainty, disorder/dispersal and information loss, and thus level of entropy, might be exacerbated or minimised. In reviewing organisational processes and practices, we ask: What contributes to increasing entropy? What contributes to minimising entropy? What are the implications for patient care?

We begin to develop understanding of entropic flow in an organisation, by interrogating circumstances (processes and practices) where tension or dysfunction is apparent (as identified by the actors involved or by knowledgeable others), and then assigning what appears to us as the most appropriate interpretation of entropy (entropic indicator) to illuminate understanding. This process of assigning entropic indicators is iterative, and involves a process of trialling interpretations and discussing these with knowledgeable others, especially the actors involved in the situation. In this way, entropic indicators can be utilised to better make sense of the causes of tension, stress or dysfunction, and identify strategic approaches for ameliorating tension.

In the two following vignettes, we demonstrate how our ComEntEth model can be engaged to foster new ways of making sense of commonly encountered circumstances in healthcare that can lead to insights about strategies to bring about improvement.

Vignette 1: Rural and remote healthcare

Synopsis

Delivery of healthcare to communities in rural and remote geographical locations, where most of the world's population live, continues to present significant challenges for policy-makers and healthcare providers. Worldwide, access is recognised as the major rural healthcare challenge. Significantly, accessing primary preventative care tends to be poorer in geographically remote populations. There are difficulties with shortages of doctors and other healthcare professionals, such as specialists, transportation to healthcare providers, communication, and infrastructure. The WHO recommends a raft of training, financial and professional development incentives to compensate healthcare practitioners for living and working in rural and remote areas (Arcury, Gesler and Preisser, 2005; McGrail and Humphreys, 2015; WHO, 2010).

Entropic indicators

Increase in entropy as *disorder/dispersal* is evident. Healthcare providers operating in spatially distanced relationships require higher energy expenditure to access other healthcare professionals and institutions, such as pathology services, diagnostic imaging and expert clinical advice. In addition, in rural settings, the energy to maintain effective coordination and connections to larger urban health services falls to fewer people, meaning many regional and remote workers must perform multiple clinical and administrative tasks that increase internal energy demands.

There is evidence of increase in *unavailability of energy*. In rural and remote areas, smaller workforces rely on multi-tasking clinical practitioners to provide both clinical and administrative expertise to sustain effective healthcare. Workers often must provide on-call, after-hours and weekend clinical and administrative services. This significantly depletes individual and collective emotional and cognitive energy to sustain healthcare services. In addition, limitations to treatment options and diagnostic services further limit the energetic inputs relied upon in modern health practices to diagnose, treat, and prevent adverse health outcomes.

Regional and remote health services increasingly rely upon short-term locum health practitioner support. The ability of short-term contract staff to build longitudinal knowledge of individual health histories, understand the limitations or pathways to accessing higher level care, and develop longer term health prevention strategies, is impacted by the loss of institutional and professional knowledge about the unique characteristics of the population and geography of regional and remote communities. This means there is evidence of increased entropy as *information loss*.

Improvement – means of ameliorating raised entropy

To minimise *disorder/dispersal* entropy, building foundations for communicative connectedness between rural and remote workers and their colleagues within other regional services and those in urban practice is necessary. This will ease some of the geographical consequences of spatial dispersion by creating opportunities for communities of practice to form across multi-disciplinary teams akin to those more easily formed around physical co-location within a large hospital setting. This can be achieved by systematic adoption of telehealth, 'virtual' medical wards with shared clinical responsibility, and access to timely specialist advice organised through formal agreement between rural and remote health services and larger urban specialist referral centres.

It is important that healthcare funders recognise the different efficiency model inherent in geographically dispersed health services so that they do not compare 'apples with oranges'. What works efficiently in urban settings may require greater funding, expertise and longer time scales to achieve in regional and remote practice. Infrastructure to support timely access to diagnostic services and larger health services, through telehealth, retrieval services, or investment in technologies such as point-of-care pathology, can reduce barriers to appropriate diagnostic and treatment outcomes for regional populations.

To address entropy as *unavailability of energy*, healthcare professionals can be enticed to rural and remote healthcare, by governing authorities offering financial and professional development incentives, such as reduction or elimination of higher education study fees or career development tied to professional training that includes early introduction to rural and remote learning opportunities. Strategies such as telehealth and service level agreements between urban and rural health districts can facilitate robust connections between remote workers and larger urban health services and thus provide quality clinical decision support. Telecommunication technologies and robust governance arrangements can bring specialised and multi-disciplinary skills and knowledge to regional and remote communities, but will also require service redesigns to ensure that rural and remote clinicians are not over burdened by additional administrative demands that increase the unavailability of their energies to perform clinical tasks.

To address entropy as *information loss*, strategies that facilitate policymakers, funders, educational institutions and professional colleges, and health service managers to work together to improve sustained retention of health workers in rural and remote areas need to be implemented. Importantly, as the quality of existing healthcare organisations within which short-term staff are employed has an impact on performance, including the quality of governance, policies and procedures for continuity of care, scope of practice, information exchange, and professional development opportunities, supporting staff to stay in areas longer, will improve the overall quality of healthcare. Staff retention fosters the opportunity for longitudinal care and more effective patient–clinician relationships which are shown to promote higher quality outcomes.

Given the influence of staffing levels, inter-professional trust, and availability of resources on clinicians' experience of psychological stress, building communicative connectedness and allocating appropriate resourcing to sustain ethical practice will benefit both the ethical context of the organisations which people create, as well as reduce the stress loads of practitioners which favours more efficient and effective clinical behaviours.

What do the entropic indicators tell us?

The entropic indicators highlight the particular issues associated with the challenges of providing rural and remote healthcare and point towards appropriate means of improvement. The entropic indicators show that energetic investments in rural and remote health are not adequate to energic needs and may increase moral stress. The above suggestions about how to reduce entropy production (as dispersal, unavailability of energy and loss of information) point to the types of investment in rural and remote healthcare that will most support rural and remote healthcare

Vignette 2: Nurse burnout/practitioner burnout

Synopsis

Health practitioner burnout is recognised as one of the key challenges in the healthcare domain across the globe. Burnout, according to the foundational research of Maslach and Leiter (1997), is characterised by emotional exhaustion, depersonalisation and reduced personal accomplishment. Maslach and Leiter describe burnout as a consequence of the prolonged mismatch between an employee and one or more of several relational dynamic factors including workload, control, reward, sense of community, fairness and personal values. The nursing profession is one particular domain in which the adverse effects of burnout have been robustly researched (Moustaka and Constantinidis, 2010). Shah et al. (2021), in a cross-sectional study of 50,000 US nurses, note that many of the complementary attributes of people who enter the nursing profession are the same factors that contribute to the experience of burnout, including motivation to care, solve problems and offer healing to those experiencing ill health, complicated by a lack of resources and inadequate support to achieve positive outcomes. Their survey found over 30% of nurses reported leaving the profession due to burnout. The potential adverse impact of nursing burnout on patients and health professionals are severe, including 'reduced job performance, poor quality of care, poor patient safety, adverse events, patient negative experience, medication errors, infections, patient falls, and intention to leave' (Dall'Ora and Saville 2021, p. 1).

Entropic indicators

Collectively, societies invest time and energy in training nursing professionals and providing the work environments in which that expertise is enlivened to provide care and recovery to suffering patients and their families. The loss of nursing professionals from clinical roles increases entropy in the form of *unavailability of energy*. This is because the energy that was previously expended in healthcare to train and sustain nurses' professional roles as anti-entropic agents is no longer available as a result of each person who leaves the profession. Overall, societies must then expend more energy to train more professionals to replace those who leave, consequently increasing entropy production across healthcare.

The link between poor patient outcomes and professional burnout is enduring. High rates of burnout increase healthcare organisation *disorder* through the introduction of avoidable harms that, but for diminished clinical performance as a result of burnout, may not otherwise have manifested. According to Panagioti et al. (2019), practitioner-induced avoidable harms may account for as much as 15% of total healthcare expenditure, meaning resources that might otherwise have been allocated to primary care and prevention are also lost, further increasing the tendency to disorder within health organisations.

Nursing effectiveness and expertise are deeply linked to the accumulation of experience over time in the healthcare setting (Hill, 2010). Entropy, as *information loss* will necessarily increase in healthcare organisations as a result of the attrition of experienced nurses from healthcare, as a consequence of burnout. However, Liao et al. (2020) suggests that burnout disproportionately affects younger nurses, meaning that over time, information loss accumulates from the failure of development of expertise amongst competently trained, but inexperienced, younger nursing professionals who leave the profession earlier.

Improvement – means of ameliorating raised entropy

Staff retention and minimisation of work related stressors, such as workload pressures, sense of control, flexible scheduling, and nurse-staffing levels, have been demonstrated as effective strategies for reducing the risk of professional burnout. In particular, a sense of control over one's job and reward for effort were found to predict less burnout in nurses (Dall'Ora and Saville, 2021).

The cumulative effect of different work related stressors results in elevated individual stress which confers a higher risk of burnout. Individual psychological stress increases the likelihood of resignation and reduced employment fraction, further depleting health system resources and thus increasing entropy across healthcare (Rees et al., 2016). In addition, moral stress has been reported as an independent factor increasing the risk of burnout amongst clinicians (Dzeng and Wachter, 2020). Rees et al. postulate that strategies aimed at improving individual mindfulness, self-efficacy and adaptive coping, can mediate psychological resilience which reduces the impact of stress and in turn the risk of burnout.

However, an emphasis on individual resilience and coping fails to consider the mechanisms via which entropy arises across organisations as complex phenomena. Weiss (2020) argues that burnout in the workplace ought to be understood as a collective issue that requires a collective response, rather than a response that relies on individuals to 'fix' the problems. From a complexity perspective, burnout is viewed as an emergent property, that arises through dynamic interactions between multiple evolving actors.

Retaining experienced nurses for longer may improve the communities of practice within which all nurses work. Hill (2010) suggests five key pillars for retention of experienced nurses: Cultivating a climate of continuous career-long learning; developing career portfolios supporting financial security; implementing ergonomic accommodations that reduce the physical burden of nursing cares; developing succession planning which enables mature, experienced staff members to work in leadership and mentoring roles; and, implementing phased retirement plans. Implementation of these strategies, we propose, would reduce entropic levels in nurses and thereby reduce burnout.

What do the entropic indicators tell us?

Entropic increase across healthcare organisations, as *unavailability of energy, disorder* and *information loss*, as a consequence of burnout amongst health professionals, particularly in the nursing discipline, significantly impacts the provision of healthcare. Both individual and collective effects of raised entropy from burnout have serious adverse consequences for the relief of suffering for patients and may cause further harm to patients and practitioners, thus contributing to the exhaustion of resources that could be otherwise directed towards restorative and anti-entropic activity within healthcare. Moderating elevated entropy from burnout requires both individual and collective adaptations to the inevitable occupational and ethical stressors arising from the nature and intensity of healthcare work.

Concluding comments

In this chapter, we interpreted organisational dynamics as entropic exchanges and investigated strategies to improve the practice of healthcare by improving entropic flow in healthcare organisations. With reference to four specific entropic indicators, we demonstrated the utility of an integrative philosophy of complexity, entropy and ethics (as depicted in our ComEntEth model), to make sense of how and why healthcare organisations promote and sustain ethical and effective modes of operating for the relief of suffering of the people they serve.

Our philosophy and theorising are situated in a conceiving of organisations that recognises both agency and structure as reciprocally shaping patterns of interaction and the daily experiences of practitioners. This characterisation preferences the importance of communicative connectedness between the actors engaged in all aspects of healthcare service: Practitioners, administrators, policy makers, and politicians. Our ComEntEth model provides a structure for discourse that becomes transdisciplinary and accessible to all actors and thereby has the capacity to facilitate growth in quotidian understanding. Takeuchi and Nonaka's organisational 'spiral' of contexts and relationships that inform organisational learning can then have a centrum in commonplace understanding around which those tasked with managing healthcare complexity might orbit.

We showed that just as suffering can be conceived as elevated entropy arising from illness and trauma in people, by necessity the organisations of healthcare, as collectives of people who create and sustain them, must manage the entropy generated by the care of the suffering, as well as the energetic transactions and transformations that power entropic exchanges between practitioners and the broader organisational milieu. Awareness of entropic reverberations across the practice of healthcare, and how to manage them, was postulated as useful in alerting practitioners, managers, administrators, funders, and policy makers about the adaptive 'self-eco-organising' of the people and organisations involved as they respond to elevated entropy and work towards the longer-term goal of a least-entropic state.

'Stress', the common vernacular for what we have termed elevated entropy, is in our characterisation, the felt-sense of increased unavailable energy, uncertainty, disorder/dispersal, and loss of information, within the individuals that constitute the practice of healthcare. Though our precis of relevant literature attests to acknowledgement of the different factors that contribute to stress in healthcare workers, we demonstrated that a unified explanatory description of these factors can be found in appreciating how they contribute to increased entropy production in practitioners. Understanding them in this way makes sense of how the factors impact on the patient and practitioner encounter at the centre of healthcare activity, with its focus on melioration of entropy in suffering patients.

In addition, we highlighted how the moral and ethical demands of clinical practice shape, and are shaped by, organisational 'ways of doing' that codify and promote certain patterns of behaviours. Unethical or morally ambiguous practices were shown to add to the stress-entropic load of practitioners and all involved in the provision of healthcare, and increase rates of burnout that contribute to unsafe patient care and poor healthcare outcomes.

Individual meliorating strategies, proposed to address stress (entropic increase) in practitioners, might be conceived of as analogous to the reciprocal and reflexive mechanisms by which biological systems adapt to, and dissipate, entropy production. In this chapter, we have highlighted the need to ensure that 'hierarchical' integrative information processing, like that of the human nervous system in individuals, is implicated in the successful management of entropy in organisations. So, rather than focus on strategies that individual practitioners might take to alleviate their workplace related sense of stress or entropic increase, we have emphasised the need for understanding of the mechanisms by which entropy manifests across an organisation.

The roles of management and leadership personnel come into focus when we consider the traditional tasks of these roles, which in thermodynamic terms can be described as 'hierarchical integrative information processing', with the potential for influencing culture and habitual ways of getting things done. However, in understanding the individual practitioners involved as rational, creative and ethical, and in taking seriously the complexity view that organisations exist as distributed sense-making capabilities of all involved, traditional roles of management and leadership can be expanded to include facilitation of opportunities to engage the distributed sense making of all involved and so build communicative connectedness. Reciprocally, coherent communicative connectedness across organisations was shown to mitigate individual stress responses.

The analysis of entropic indicators in the two vignettes presented in this chapter reminds us that, successful responses to rising entropy involve distributed and formally organised mechanisms for communicative connectedness, autonomy, control, and creative thinking, that allow different agencies to define and solve the infinite problems of the micro-state potentialities of practice, to ensure optimised macro-state organisational outcomes of safe, effective, and efficient care.

References

Arcury, T., Gesler, W. and Preisser, J. (2005) 'The Effects of Geography and Spatial Behaviour on Health Care Utilisation Among the Residents of a Rural Region'. *Health Services Research.* 40(1):135–156.

Atabay, G., Cangarli, B. and Penbek, S. (2015) 'Impact of Ethical Climate on Moral Distress Revisited: Multidimensional View'. *Nursing Ethics.* 22(1):103–116.

Australian Medical Association (AMA) (2011) *Position Statement: Health and Well-Being of Doctors and Medical Students.* AMA.

Bartholdson, C., Sandeberg, K., Lutzen, K., Blomgren, K. and Perget, P. (2016) 'Healthcare Professionals' Perceptions of the Ethical Climate in Paediatric Cancer Care.' *Nursing Ethics.* 23(8):877–888.

Berland, A., Natvig, G. K. and Gundersen, D. (2008) 'Patient Safety and Job Related Stress: A Focus Group Study'. *Intensive and critical care nursing.* 24(2):90–97.

Bienertova-Vasku, J., Zlamal, F., Necesanek, I., Konecny, D. and Vasku, A. (2016) 'Calculating Stress: From Entropy to a Thermodynamic Concept of Health and Disease'. *PLOS One.* 11:1.

Blons, E., Arsac, L. M., Gilfriche, P., McLeod, H., Lespinet-Najib, V., Grivel, E. and Deschodt-Arsac, V. (2019) 'Alterations in Heart-Brain Interactions Under Mild Stress During a Cognitive Task Are Reflected in Entropy of Heart Rate Dynamics'. *Scientific Reports*. 9:18190.

British Medical Association (BMA) (2000) *Work Related Stress Among Senior Doctors: Review of Research*. London: BMA.

Brunero, S., Cowan, D., Grochulski, A. and Garvey, A. (2006) *Stress Management for Nurses*. Camperdown: New South Wales Nurses' Association.

Clausius, R. (1867) *The Mechanical Theory of Heat, With Its Applications to the Steam Engine and to the Physical Properties of Bodies* (T. Archer Hirst, Ed). London: J. Van Voorst.

Clegg, S., Kornberger, M. and Pitsis, T. (2005) *Managing and Organisations: An Introduction to Theory and Practice*. London: Sage.

Dall'Ora, C. and Saville, C. (2021) 'Burnout in Nursing: What Have We Learnt and What Is Still Unknown?'. *Nursing Times*. 117(2):43–44.

Dewa, C. S., Loong, D., Bonata, S. and Trojanowski, L. (2017) 'The Relationship between Physician Burnout and Quality of Healthcare in Terms of Safety and Acceptability: A Systematic Review'. *British Medical Journal Open*. 7:e015141. doi:10.1136/bmjopen-2016-015141

Dieser, R. B., Edginton, C. R. and Ziemer, R. (2017) 'Decreasing Patient Stress and Physician/Medical Workforce Burnout Through Health Care Environments: Uncovering the Serious Leisure Perspective at Mayo Clinic's Campus in Rochester, Minnesota'. *Mayo Clinic Proceedings*. 92(7):1080–1087.

Dzeng, E. and Wachter, R. M. (2020) 'Ethics in Conflict: Moral Distress as a Root Cause of Burnout'. *Journal of General Internal Medicine*. 35:409–411.

Elias, N. (1978) *The Civilising Process, Vol. 1: The History of Manners* (Edmund Jephcott, Trans). New York: Urizen Books.

Familoni, O. (2008) 'An Overview of Stress in Medical Practice'. *African Health Sciences*. 8(1):6–7.

Fimian, M. J., Lieberman, R. J. and Fastenau, P. S. (Apr. 1991) 'Development and Validation of an Instrument to Measure Occupational Stress in Speech-Language Pathologists'. *Journal of Speech, Language and, Hearing Research*. 34(2):439–446.

Giddens, A. (1971) *Capitalism and Modern Social Theory*. Cambridge University Press: London.

Giffin, B. J., Purcell, N., Burkman, K., Litz, B. T., Bryan, C. J., Schmitz, M., Villierme, C. Walsh, J. and Maguen, S. (2019) 'Moral Injury: An Integrative Review'. *Journal of Traumatic Stress*. 32:350–362.

Grey, C. (2005) *A Very Short, Fairly Interesting and Reasonably Cheap Book About Studying Organizations*. London: Sage.

Hill, K. (2010) 'Improving quality and patient safety by retaining nursing expertise.' *Online Journal of Issues in Nursing*. 15:1–9.

Hogarth, R. M. (2010) 'Intuition: A challenge for psychological research on decision making'. *Psychological Inquiry*. 21(4):338–353.

Koinis, A., Giannou, V., Drantaki, V., Angelaina, S., Stratou, E. and Saridi, M. (Apr. 13, 2015) 'The Impact of Healthcare Workers Job Environment on Their

Mental-emotional Health. Coping strategies: The Case of a Local general Hospital'. *Health Psychology Research*. 3(1).

Kumar, S. (Sep. 2016) 'Burnout and Doctors: Prevalence, Prevention and Intervention'. *Healthcare (Basel)*. 4(3):37.

Liao, R, Yeh, M. Lin, K. and Wang, K. (2020) 'A hierarchical model of occupational burnout in nurses associated with job-induced stress, self-concept and work environment.' *Journal of Nurse Research*. April:28(2).

Lindsay, R., Hanson, L., Taylor, M. and McBurney, H. (2008) 'Workplace Stressors Experienced by Physiotherapists Working in Regional Public Hospitals'. *The Australian Journal of Rural Health*. 16(4):187–251.

Maslach, C. and Leiter, M. P. (1997) *The truth about burnout: How organisations cause personal stress and what to do about it.* New Jersey: Jossey-Bass.

McGrail, M. and Humphreys, J. (Nov. 4, 2015) 'Spatial Access Disparities to Primary Health Care in Rural and Remote Australia'. *Geospat Health*. 10(2):358.

Melucci, A. (1996) *The Playing Self.* Cambridge: Cambridge University Press.

Moustaka, E. and Constantinidis, T. (2010) 'Sources and Effects of Work-Related Stress in Nursing'. *Health Science Journal*. 4:4.

Nalliah, R. P. (2016) 'Clinical Decision Making: Choosing Between Intuition, Experience and Scientific Evidence'. *British Dental Journal*. 221:752–754.

Nelson, W. A., Gardent, P. B., Shulman, E. and Splaine, M. E. (2010) 'Preventing Ethics Conflicts and Improving Healthcare Quality Through System Redesign'. *Quality and Safety in Healthcare*. 19(6):526–530.

Pakhomov, A. and Sudin, N. (2013) 'Thermodynamic View on Decision-Making Process: Emotions as a Potential Power Vector of Realization of the Choice'. *Cognition Neurodynamic*. 7(6):449–463.

Panagioti, M., Khan, K., Keers, R. N., Abuzour, A., Phipps, D., Kontopantellis, E., Bower, P., Campbell, S., Haneef, R. Avery, A. J. and Ashcroft, D. (2019) 'Prevalence, severity, and nature of preventable patient harm across medical care settings: Systematic review and meta-analysis.' *British Medical Journal*. 366:4185.

Peters, A., McEwen, B. S. and Friston, K. (2017) 'Uncertainty and Stress: Why It Causes Diseases and How It Is Mastered by the Brain'. *Progress in Neurobiology*. 156:164–188.

Riley, R., Spiers, J., Buszewicz, M., Taylor, A., Thornton, G. and Chew-Graham, C. (2018) 'What Are the Sources of Stress and Distress for General Practitioners Working in England? A Qualitative Study'. *British Medical Journal Open*. 8(1):e017361. doi:10.1136/bmjopen-2017-017361

Rees, C. S., Heritage, B., Osseiran-Moisson, R., Chamberlain, D., Cusack, L., Anderson, J., Terry, V., Rogers, C. Hemsworth, D., Cross and Hegney, D. G. (2016) 'Can we predict burnout among student nurses? An exploration of the ACWR-1 model of individual psychological resilience.' *Frontiers in Psychology*. 19 July 2019.

Rongjun, Y. (2016) 'Stress Potentiates Decision Biases: A Stress Induced-Deliberation-to-Intuition (SIDI) Model'. *Neurobiology of Stress*. 3:83–95.

Shah, M., K., Gandrakota, N., Cimiotti, J. P., Ghose, N., Moore, M. and Ali, M. K. (2021) 'Prevalence of and factors Associated with Nurse Burnout in the US'. *JAMA Netw Open*. 4:2.

Shannon, C. E. (1948) 'A Mathematical Theory of Communication'. *Bell System Technology Journal.* 27(3):379–423.

Silva, D. S., Gibson, J. L., Sibbald, R., Connolly, E. and Singer, P. A. (2008) 'Clinical Ethicists' Perspectives on Organisational Ethics in Healthcare Organisations'. *Journal of Medical Ethics.* 35(5):320–323.

Stacey, R. (2000) 'Organisations as Complex Responsive Processes of Relating'. *Journal of Innovative Management.* 8(2):27–39.

Stacey, R. D. (2002/2003) 'Organisations as Complex Responsive Processes of Relating'. Journal of Innovative Management. 8(2):27–39.

Stacey, R. D., Griffin, D. and Shaw, P. (2000) *Complexity and Management.* London: Routledge.

Stebbins, R. A. (1982) 'Serious Leisure: A Conceptual Statement'. *Pacific Sociological Review.* 25(2):251–272.

Takeuchi, H. and Nonaka, I. (2004) *Theory of Organisational Knowledge Creation.* New Jersey: John Wiley and Sons.

Tinley, P. (2015) 'Occupational Stress Among Australia Podiatrists in General and Geriatric Practice'. *Journal of Foot and Ankle Research.* 8:16.

Ulrich, C., Taylor, C. and Penbek, S. (2013) 'Everyday Ethics: Ethical Issues and Stress in Nursing Practice'. *Journal of Advanced Nursing.* 66(11):2510–2519.

Vickers, G. (1984) *Human Systems are Different.* London: Harper and Row.

Weber, M. (1947) *The Theory of Social and Economic Organisation* (A. M. Henderson and Talcott Parsons, Trans). London: Macmillan Publishers.

Weiss, L. (2020) 'Burnout from an organisational perspective.' *Stanford Social Innovation Review.* https://doi.org/10.48558/6CVo-C436.

Wenger, E. (1998) *Communities of Practice.* Cambridge: Cambridge University Press.

West, M. and Coia, D. (2019) *Caring for Doctors, Caring for Patients.* General Medical Council UK.

World Medical Association Statement on Physicians Well-being (2015) www.wma.net/policies-post/wma-statement-on-physicians-well-being/

World Health Organization (2010) *Increasing Access to Health Workers in Remote and Rural Areas Through Improved Retention: Global Policy Recommendations.* ISBN. 978 92 4 1156401 1.

4 Entropy and Healthcare in a Pandemic

Introduction

Pandemics, infectious diseases that spread rapidly across large regions, affecting many people (Morens, Folkers and Fauci, 2009), devastate lives, societies, healthcare organisations, industries, economies, governments, and countries. In the context of the WHO's warning that with intense human mobility, pandemics are spreading faster and further (WHO, 2018), in this chapter, we utilise our ComEntEth (Complex Entropic Ethical) model to identify principles for optimising the capacity of healthcare organisations to provide safe and effective care during and after pandemics.

We frame pandemics as constituting an explosive increase of entropy production in individuals and societies across the globe. Consideration of SARS-CoV-2 in terms of increase in entropy production fosters an appreciation of the rapid entropic increase of suffering as disease and as fear, disruption and stress across society.

In this chapter, we critically examine the self-organisation, dynamism and emergence of governing authority, societal and healthcare responses to the SARS-CoV-2 pandemic, with reference to entropic transactions. We explain how the pandemic induces rapid increase in entropy that threatens overall viability of individuals, healthcare organisations and the broader societal environments within which they are situated. We highlight the centrality of an ethics of responsibility to the responses of government, society and healthcare organisations and identify principles for activating effective preventative and restorative processes for lowering entropic increase in countries, societies, communities and healthcare organisations.

ComEntEth model: A theoretical framework for understanding and informing responses to a pandemic

As detailed in previous chapters, we draw on the complexity sciences, thermodynamics (the concept of entropy) and ethics (Levinas's ethics of

DOI: 10.4324/9781003197454-4

responsibility) to propose a philosophical grounding for healthcare. In this section, we briefly outline the major tenants of our ComEntEth model to point towards how it can inform strategies for responding to a pandemic, and in so doing, improve global health security.

A complexity paradigm explores the dynamics of phenomena of the world as self-organising, dynamic and emergent (Kuhn, 2009). Pandemics and human responses can be understood to conform with complexity principles: They too emerge through self-organising, dynamic, interconnected processes.

Consideration of these processes as entropic exchanges and transformations elaborates understanding of the structure of living entities and the mechanisms by which they resist decay (Morin, 2008; Prigogine, 1980). Pandemics manifest rapid increase in entropy production in individuals and across countries, that threaten individual and collective viability. Analysis of circumstances and mechanisms whereby entropic manifestation, as unavailable energy, uncertainty, disorder/dispersal, and information loss, and thus levels of entropy, might be exacerbated or minimised, provides useful information about effective strategies to control the effects of a pandemic.

Levinas's ethics of relationship offers an ethical basis for the power of suffering to elicit in others a desire to give relief from suffering (Levinas, 2003). Global and local responses to management of a pandemic attest to an ethics of responsibility to prevent or reduce the suffering of others.

Thus, our ComEntEth framework theorises responses to a pandemic as energetic relational exchanges between complex, self-organising, dynamic and emergent phenomenon, where the exchanges unfold around a central attractor: Minimisation of the suffering or rapid entropic increase associated with a pandemic. This explanation is understood to hold across scale, from the genetic to the biological and social.

In principle, whether between patient and healthcare practitioner, or practitioner and healthcare organisation, minimisation of entropy is understood to be achieved by entropic exchanges with the surrounding system/environment. In thermodynamic terms, for this to occur effectively, the system under review (patient, healthcare organisation, national healthcare organisation) requires its environment to have the capacity to provide the energy necessary to minimise entropic increase.

With a pandemic, we can expect widespread elevation in entropy production, across individuals, societies and healthcare organisations, which means the capacity of surrounding environments to provide energy may be severely impacted. It is important, therefore, to explore the strategies employed by governments and societal and healthcare organisations to minimise the increased entropy production associated with a pandemic, in the context of worldwide entropic increase.

We propose that our ComEntEth framework provides a means of interrogating and extending understanding of (1) the strategies employed by an array of agencies (government, social and organisational) tasked with responding to the COVID-19 pandemic, and (2) the means via which human society might better protect itself from the health impact and social-economic disruption of a pandemic.

What is known about the process of emergence of a pandemic

While we cannot predict the nature of the virus, source or place of outbreak, with the continued intensity of human-animal contact and mobility of human populations, we can expect pandemics to emerge from time to time (WHO, 2018). The WHO advises that at a macro level, when a pandemic emerges there will be (1) an initial delay in recognition; (2) enormous impact on day to day habits of living; (3) social reactions of fear, confusion and refusal to acknowledge its existence and (4) amplification of reactions via media coverage. These responses all signify increase in entropy production.

Local self-organising interrelationships responses and dynamics (of countries, cultures, geographies) mean that the pandemic will unfold differently in different parts of the world. However, as research into previous epidemics and pandemics has shown, the dynamics of the evolution of a pandemic typically occur in four phases: (1) Introduction in a community; (2) Localised transmission of pathogens; (3) Amplification as the pathogen rapidly spreads across vast regions and populations; and (4) Reduced transmission due to acquired population immunity, elimination or eradication (WHO, 2018). Described in terms of increase in entropy production, these phases can be depicted as: Rapid increase in entropy in a few individuals; rapid increase in entropy of groups of people within certain communities; rapidly escalating increase in entropy (as disease, fear, disruption and stress) across vast regions and populations; and, reduction in pandemic related entropy production.

The WHO proposes that a sequence of interventions in response to these phases is necessary to limit growth of the pandemic. Schematically, the phases, interventions and indicative entropic production can be depicted as shown in Figure 4.1.

Using these known parameters, in the following sections, we explore in broad outline, indicative government and social responses to the SARS-CoV-2 pathogen, demonstrating how these shape healthcare responses. Recognising interrelatedness between the government, societal norms and expectations, and healthcare organisations of a country or territory, this exploration is intended to provide a context for subsequent exploration of healthcare responses.

Phase/*entropy*	Intervention
1. Introduction or emergence [entropy+]	Anticipation and early detection
2. Localised transmission [entropy++]	Containment
3. Amplification [entropy+++]	Control and mitigation
4. Reduced transmission/immunity [entropy-]	Elimination or eradication

Figure 4.1 WHO phases, interventions and entropic production

Government and societal responses to the process of emergence of the SARS-CoV-2 Virus (COVID-19)

We survey government and social responses to SARS-CoV-2 (the virus that causes the disease COVID-19) and its management, in accord with the WHO's four phases of evolution of a pandemic and associated responses. In so doing, we draw on our ComEntEth model to inform understanding and identify the attractors guiding choices.

The emergence of a new viral pandemic implicates multiple variables, from the biological to the social, political, economic and geographic and can be traced back to relationships between constituent parts, be these cells, bodies, communities, societies and their various governing bodies, that evolve over time as they interact and influence one another, giving rise to emergent collective behaviours (such as spread of COVID-19, management strategies of leaders and revolts against containment directives). A complexity perspective forewarns to expect contingency and uncertainty as individuals, countries, territories and groups emerge concurrently. Recognising that what is known is constantly shifting, and complete knowledge is not possible, a complexity perspective is useful in discerning underlying patterns of order and attractors that inform about the processes of emergence.

Phase 1: Introduction (anticipatory and early detection responses)

In December 2019, patients presented at the Wuhan Central Hospital, Hubei, China, with pneumonia of an unknown cause. On 31 December, 2019, the Wuhan Municipal Health Commission reported 'a cluster of cases of pneumonia' to the WHO (WHO, 2020a). On 1 January, 2020, the WHO set up an Incident Management Support Team (IMST) across its organisation (headquarters, regional headquarters and country level). The WHO reported the outbreak on social media (4 January) and via a technical publication, 'Disease Outbreak News', on 5 January, 2020. At this time Chinese authorities were strictly managing the information that could be released about this new potential pandemic.

At a macro level, this initial emergence of a new pneumonia involved just three variables – the new pathogen, Chinese citizens, and the WHO. As French mathematician Henri Poincare (Coveney and Highfield, 1996) showed in the nineteenth century, with as few as three variables we should expect complex behaviour that is difficult to describe and where the initial conditions will significantly influence future emergence.

This beginning to the pandemic is as predicted by the WHO. At first, only a small number of people in a specific area were affected and the sense that SARS-CoV-2 constituted a potential pandemic was not yet generally appreciated. The actions of the Chinese government to restrict sharing of information about the existence of this new SARS disease can be understood as a way of minimising widespread social fear and disruption, and hence rise in entropy. However, as social media and press reports began to circulate on the existence of a new and dangerous disease, the lack of information sharing from Chinese authorities only added to uncertainty and concern (and hence entropic rise) across the globe. The Wuhan Municipal Health Commission's reporting of the outbreak to the WHO and the WHO's subsequent actions, including setting up the IMST, and publishing the first Disease Outbreak News on this new virus, provide evidence of global and local anticipatory and early detection strategies.

Expressed in thermodynamic terms, the motivation to act in response to SARS-CoV-2 was activated by a felt sense of rising entropy, anticipatory fear and uncertainty, and lack of knowledge about the potential of the new virus to cause world-wide havoc. The actions of the Chinese authorities to report and minimise sharing of information, indicate responses designed to minimise entropic increase (as uncertainty, lack of knowledge and the need to re-organise). The WHO's actions can be interpreted as a deliberate and necessary means of alerting regions and countries beyond Wuhan, to a potential new threat, a deliberate perturbation to homeostatic conditions in countries, agencies and healthcare organisations across the globe.

Expressed in terms of Levinas's conceptualisation of self-other responsibility, both the Chinese authorities' and the WHO's responses can be viewed as motivated by a desire to minimise and protect people from the suffering of disease and social/economic upheaval.

Phase 2: Localised transmission (containment measures)

With the detection of the cluster of pneumonia cases of an unknown aetiology, the Communist Party of China, Central Committee and the Chinese State Council launched a nation emergency response and instigated measures.

Their containment strategies sought to control the source of infection, block transmission and prevent further spread from Wuhan. Wet markets were closed, work began on identification of the zoonotic source, and the Chinese government continued to work closely with the WHO.

By 12 January 2020, scientists had recognised the pathogen's similarity to the SARS virus of 2003, sequenced its genome and named the virus SARS-CoV-2 (WHO, 2020b). That scientists so quickly identified the genomic sequencing of the pathogen responsible for SARS-CoV-2, indicates global authority, and country level, preparedness and anticipation.

Research, such as genomic sequencing, signifies the beginning of activities that seek to contain the virus outbreak and to restore homeostasis of individuals with COVID-19, and prevent future perturbation of SARS-CoV-2, to social, economic and healthcare homeostasis. Homeostasis in this usage refers to how individuals and human collectives (such as societies or healthcare organisations) can maintain stable conditions despite competing political, economic, cultural and so on, pressures.

The Chinese containment measures comprised proactive surveillance enabling early case detection, rapid diagnosis and case isolation, limitations to social gathering, and rigorous tracking and quarantine of close contacts. According to the WHO, in a remarkably short time frame, the Chinese scientists and health experts 'isolated the causative virus, established diagnostic tools, and determined key transmission parameters, such as the route of spread and incubation period' (WHO, 2020a, p. 17).

It is evident that the significant initial conditions for the success of the Chinese governing bodies' SARS-CoV-2 containment strategies, lies with the compliance and commitment of the Chinese citizens to collective action to contain the virus.

High levels of communicative connectedness and trust, also in evidence, support compliance, collective commitment and the capacity of the Chinese society to contain the spread of SARS-CoV-2. The communally felt uncertainty (and associated entropic increase) surrounding the virus was mitigated both through the rapidity with which the Chinese authorities gained necessary information about cause, diagnosis and transmission, and by their daily sharing of information with the Chinese people.

Although these early containment strategies were energy consuming, they served to limit long term elevation in entropy that would arise from increasing spread of illness, and radical and ongoing need for re-organisation.

Phase 3: Amplification (control and mitigation)

Just as the first wave of COVID-19 was being contained in China, the disease was rapidly spreading across the world. The WHO advised on

30 January that SARS-CoV-2 constituted a Public Health Emergency of International Concern (PHEIC). However, it was only following continued rapid spread and severity of the disease, in concert with 'alarming levels of inaction' and ambivalence about implementing restrictive interventions by countries across the world, that WHO advised, on 11 March, 2020, that COVID-19 be characterised as a pandemic (WHOb, 2020).

The WHO counsels that once the disease is recognised as a pandemic, the goal should be to 'mitigate its impact and reduce its incidence, morbidity and mortality, as well as disruptions to economic, political and social systems (2018, p. 30). While mitigation efforts require energy (and thus raise entropy levels), they serve to reduce widespread and long-term entropy increase (as associated with illness and the stress of economic, political and social disruption).

Somewhere between the local transmission phase and this amplification phase, countries and governments outside China, were required to respond to the WHO and other scientific consensus that the local containment strategies within the Chinese state had not successfully mitigated the spread of the virus from Hubei and surrounding provinces. Against this background, it is of interest to explore indications of the diversity of country responses to the SARS-CoV-2 pandemic.

The complexity concept of 'sensitive dependence on initial conditions' highlights how the initial conditions prevalent in a country when the pandemic first arrives significantly shapes management of the spread of SARS-CoV-2. We consider something of the initial conditions at play, by surveying the major strategies employed by governing authorities to manage entropic increase and reflecting on the role of communicative connectedness in supporting a 'whole of society' response to management of the SARS-CoV-2 pandemic. Exploring some of the emblematic strategies employed by different nations in response to rising entropy at this early stage of development, can offer useful insights into how sensitivity to initial conditions can in complex phenomena, result in divergent macro-states over time.

Initial conditions

The initial conditions for each country vary and include government attitudes, social and cultural norms, attitudes towards those in authority, relationships between various levels of governance, national wealth, capacity of the healthcare system, social mobility and experience of, and preparedness for, dealing with a major health crisis. Domestic factors such as these are juxtaposed to a backdrop of shared opportunity to make sense of the information provided by leading healthcare organisations about management of local transmission and early amplification of the viral vector and its subsequent illness.

Reflecting on the range of initial responses to evidence of a viral pandemic, we identify three characteristic attitudes in play that shaped societal and government narratives about the pandemic and responses to it: (1) Dismissal – Nothing to see here, (2) Complacency – It'll be alright and (3) Alarm – It's a pandemic. Each of these attitudes can be linked to choices made about control and mitigation responses as cases of COVID-19 began to exponentially increase across countries. With so much in flux as the pandemic emerged (and continues to evolve), we see these attitudes not as stable fixed points, but as indicative of early responses. As the various control and mitigation measures were implemented, a fourth characteristic attitude linked most strongly with citizens and social groups became apparent: (4) Revolt – You can't control me.

The triggering event energising a response to the pandemic can be understood to arise from a change in the steady state of the individual or social structure. The change in steady state establishes a tension that requires a response within the organism or society, and/or alterations to the surrounding environment, to resolve and re-establish order. In short, it is our proposition that the motivation to act is triggered by rising entropy which is sensed within the individual or society as a threat that may lead to disintegration or dissolution, as steady states of organisation begin to shift or collapse.

Recourse to the first three indicative characteristic attitudes shows how the initial responses of a country shape efforts to control and mitigate the spread of COVID-19, and by extension, the preparedness and capacity of healthcare organisations to meet the demands of the pandemic.

The first response, *Dismissal – Nothing to see here*, signifies an active oppositional stance that dismisses news of the COVID-19 pandemic. Despite the WHO's notifications of 4 and 5 January alerting countries to the threat of SARS-CoV-2 and the need for implementation of restrictive measures, together with its 11 March announcement that SARS-CoV-2 constituted a pandemic, some continued to dismiss the seriousness of the threat. For example:

> In my understanding the destructive power of this virus is over estimated. Maybe it's even being promoted for economic reasons.
> (Jair Bolsonaro, Brazil President, 9 March, 2020)

> We, the poor, are immune to the coronavirus.
> (Miguel Angel Barbosa, Governor,
> Puebla, Mexico, March, 2020).

Although not alone, the US President Donald Trump exemplified this attitude. A few weeks after the WHO and Chinese authorities had issued worldwide alerts about the seriousness of the SARS-CoV-2 pathogen, the first confirmed US case of COVID-19 was declared on 21 January, 2020. Asked by a CNBC reporter on 22 January about the virus spreading in the US, President Trump responded:

> We have it totally under control. It's one person coming in from China . . . It's going to be just fine.
>
> (US President Trump, January, 2021)

Despite this attitude, on 3 February, the broader US administration declared a public health emergency and commenced a raft of social and health policy initiatives to contain the spread of the virus in the US.

Nevertheless, as expert members of the US National Institutes of Health and the Centers for Disease Control and Prevention (CDC) report, President Trump and his administration 'silenced scientists, meddled in their reports and ignored their advice' (Viglione, 2020). The Select Subcommittee on the Coronavirus Crisis reported at least 47 instances of political interference by President Trump and his administrative officials, between February and September 2020, 'overruling and sidelining top scientists and undermining American's health to advance the president's partisan agenda' (2020, p. 1).

On this background, cases continue to surge in the US. The CDC notes over 76.2 million infections and more than 900,000 deaths from COVID-19 (February 5, 2022), with community transmission classified as high (CDC, 2022).

Healthcare organisations across the US reported alarming inadequacy of supply of Personal Protective Equipment (PPE), ventilators, healthcare workers and coordinated preparedness to meet the dramatically escalating demands to manage the pandemic health impacts (Ranney, Griffeth and Jha, 2020). Given the role of the US Federal Government, the Trump Administration's intransigent adherence to the dismissal narrative likely directly impacted the capacity of healthcare in the US to meet the sudden urgent demands created by the pandemic during the amplification phase.

President Trump and his administration's publicly presented attitude of dismissal can be interpreted as a means to limit increase in entropy by seeking to limit fear and uncertainty. In contradistinction, being at odds with senior health authority's advice, it also served to increase uncertainty and so increase entropy.

By insisting that business as usual was the appropriate response, given the position that no threat existed, governments that took this stance reinforced normal modes of activity to maintain relations between citizens. However, this approach also prevented quick dissemination of information and encouragement of citizens to comply with mitigation strategies.

The second response, *Complacency – It'll be alright*, assumes that with time and minimum interruption to normal activities, the spread and severity of the pandemic will subside. For example:

> We believe the risk of a global pandemic is very much upon us and as a result, as a government, we need to take the steps necessary to prepare for such a pandemic. . . . There is no need for us to be moving to having mass gatherings of people stop. . . . You can still go to the football and the cricket and play with your friends down the street.
>
> (Australian Prime Minister Scott Morrison, 27 February, 2021)

In Australia, this attitude was evidenced in some of the Federal Government responses (as aforementioned) and in a proportion of the population. Despite these early political assurances, as the dramatic changing circumstances of the pandemic continued and more restrictive measures were recommended, most Australians appeared to 'do the right thing', by following COVID-19 advice (Seale et al., 2020). However, some citizens repeatedly, and deliberately, ignored the advice. Non-adherence to strict isolation guidelines resulted in multiple failures of quarantine and led inevitably, to increasing numbers of COVID-19 cases, in tandem with States and Territories changing the 'advice' to 'rules', increasing the specificity of limitations and increasing penalties for non-compliance. Complacency is demonstrated by families, who during periods of lockdown, continued to hold large family events. As Victorian Premier Daniel Andrews notes, 'the [COVID-19] numbers are being driven by families . . . having big get-togethers and not following the advice around social distancing' (Tsirtsakis, 2020). Similarly, it is evidenced by large crowds gathering at popular beaches, such as Bondi, and completely ignoring stay-at-home and social distancing rules, creating events that formed 'super spreader' conditions for infection amplification.

The failure by the Australian Federal Government to procure sufficient Pfizer vaccine, and the over reliance on local production of the AstraZeneca vaccine, further evidences a degree of complacency. Prime Minister Morrison's infamous claim that the vaccine rollout is 'not a race' is indicative of this complacent attitude. While other countries were lobbying Pfizer to ensure adequate supplies of the vaccine, following Pfizer's June 2020 suggestion of a meeting with the Federal Health Minister Greg Hunt and senior departmental executives, a health department first assistant secretary, Lisa Schofield, instead attended the meeting (Martin, 2021).

The Australian Federal Government's early responses to the SARS-CoV-2 were in part shaped by low numbers of COVID-19 cases in Australia compared with other places such as Europe, the US, the UK, and the South Americas. The felt level of entropic increase, associated with potential suffering from disease was not sufficient for the whole population to willingly accept restrictions that interfered with their lifestyle, nor for the Federal Government to instigate with some urgency, proactive measures such as procurement of adequate vaccine supplies.

The third response, *Alarm – It's a pandemic*, was evidenced in scientists, medical professionals, some governments, and citizens dispersed across the world, in those who recognised the pandemic potential of SARS-CoV-2 and advocated that governments and societies immediately attend to preparedness plans in readiness.

Perhaps most demonstrative of an 'alarmist' reaction was that of the Hong Kong Special Administrative Region of the People's Republic of China. Hong Kong had suffered severe social, economic, and health impacts from the 2003 SARS epidemic and following this, created the Center for Health Protection (CHP) which is responsible for responding to all infectious diseases. With the first confirmed case of COVID-19, the government instigated 'emergency' level actions, such as strict border control, quarantine measures, testing, and contact tracing. Citizens were asked to social distance, wear masks and be vigilant about personal and environmental hygiene. Sophia Chan, Hong Kong's Secretary for Food and Health considers that because of the country's experience with SARS in 2003, there was a high level of government and social proactivity and diligence that created strong mitigation and control measures against the spread of SARS-CoV-2 (Chan, 2020).

Higher levels of entropy are associated with uncertainty. In Hong Kong, there appears to be low levels of uncertainty (and hence low entropy) in relation to the outbreak of the COVID-19 pandemic. This can be attributed to a number of factors, including, the high level of trust and coherence between the people and the government, early imposition of protective control measures and the readiness of the Hong Kong people to comply with these and maintain personal diligence. There was also in evidence a strong cultural sense of self-other responsibility, with people highly conscious of not wanting to affect other people nor put them at risk (Saiidi, 2020).

Ensuing government and social responses

As SARS-CoV-2 spread globally, most countries instituted comprehensive measures such as border closures, physical distancing, stay at home orders, mask wearing and attention to personal hygiene, to slow its spread and thus reduce mortality and morbidity, and prevent overwhelm of healthcare services.

Across the world, as images and stories of individual suffering, overwhelmed hospitals and mass graves were disseminated, the severity of the threat of COVID-19 became real to citizens, even in countries where the virus was yet to escalate. This instigated more active government and social responses. Contemporary technology and social media in this regard were critical to keeping people across the world informed, safe and connected, and thereby assisting in limiting the entropic increase of disease and social and economic disruption, via dissemination of useful information, that is, anti-entropic information.

The specifics of government responses and compliance rates of citizens varied across different countries and states. In Hungary, for example, Prime Minister Viktor Orban included in his 'Draft Law on Protecting Against Coronavirus' that anyone who spread 'distorted truths' about the virus, or interferes with the 'implementation of epidemiological isolation' would be punished with prison time (Zerofsky, 2020). In contrast, the Swedish government based its response on recognising the individual responsibility of citizens to stay home when they have symptoms. The Swedish Public Health Agency (FHM) initially employed a de-facto herd immunity approach that allowed community transmission to occur with little mandatory social isolation measures in place. Over time, however, incremental restrictive interventions have been introduced (Claeson and Hanson, 2020).

In countries such as Australia and the US, the response involved both federal and state governments, with at times tensions between these governing authorities. In the US, with the federal government responsible for funding scientific and medical research into testing, treatment and vaccines, and state governments responsible for containment, testing and treatment responses, state lockdowns can be understood to be related to the availability of adequate testing, treatment and vaccine options (Bergquist, Otten and Sarich, 2020). Beyond these factors, with isolation and lockdown measures evolving out of myriad interactions between federal and state authorities, influenced by political persuasions and prevailing local conditions, responses vary from state to state.

In tandem with restrictive actions, governments around the world, along with the WHO, utilised contemporary technological capacities and social media to provide citizens with up-to-date information, not only about the spread of COVID-19, but also about strategies to stay safe, including information on where to get tested, and local physical isolation rules. In Australia, each State utilised television and a range of social media channels, to publish up-to-date local and global COVID-19 information. These daily reports included detail about numbers, age groups and vaccination status of people infected or who have died within each 24-hour period, specific COVID-19 infection sites and updates on COVID-19 rules and restrictions.

This information sharing served a number of purposes. On the one hand, by including details of cases and deaths, as well as condolence messages, the messaging tended to keep entropic increase associated with fear of catching the disease at an elevated state. This served to encourage citizens and organisations to be vigilant in their COVID safe behaviours. On the other hand, the daily reports served to halt the entropic increase of stress and fear, by assuring citizens of the requisite capacity of the governing authorities and medical experts to keep people safe and manage the consequences of amplification.

The range of the ensuing responses to management of SARS-CoV-2 demonstrates something of the complexity of the pandemic and responses to it. They indicate the influence of initial conditions on the subsequent evolution of the disease trajectory, along with the interdependency between the pandemic, and social and governing responses. The various responses indicate increased entropy production as individuals, societies and governments expended energy in grappling with uncertainty, re-organisation of social structures and habits of living and lack of information. The suffering of others and a sense of 'self-other' responsibility, whereby 'their suffering could be mine' can be seen as the major attractor motivating government and social actions to mitigate the spread of SARS-CoV-2.

Lockdowns are enormously disruptive. Severe restrictions on movement, consumption, and the rhythms of daily life, grossly distort and halt the normal economic behaviours of industry and consumers, triggering disastrous effects (also manifest as entropic rise) across the tightly integrated domestic and international economies of the world. Consumer, corporate and global trade are all affected by global supply chain disruptions, compression of demand and macroeconomic instability. The public debt of countries across the world has risen sharply as a consequence of government expenditure to support incomes, along with loss of tax revenue as economic activity diminished. These effects indicate how COVID-19 has realised economically related entropic increase and thus negative impact on human societies (Hidayat, Farooq and Alim, 2020).

Indicative of the felt sense of entropic elevation, the sustained conditions of limitations to daily rhythms, loss of income and social isolation affected the mental health of individuals across countries. A systematic review in *The Lancet* reported major increases in depression and anxiety disorders associated with countries and regions of the world with the highest daily infection and death rates. An additional 52 million people are estimated to have suffered depression and anxiety disorders (an indication of entropic increase) attributable to COVID-19, with psychological effects particularly acute for patients and healthcare professionals in direct contact with the outbreak (Santomauro, 2021).

A range of alternative misinformation narratives emerged in certain sectors of societies, where there was not the requisite trust in authorities, nor the educational experience necessary to grasp the medical explanations about COVID-19, its treatment and mitigation of spread. For example, as a medical doctor, one of us (Le Plastrier), recalls patients repeatedly asking him if breathing techniques, lemon juice, and herbal supplements, being promulgated as a reliable defence against COVID-19, were true. The source of those claims was a Facebook post purporting to have been created by a 'Chinese scientist' who had studied the effects of the virus in China during the early pandemic. Similarly, in India, 'consuming cow urine and Gangaajal (water of the Ganga river), clapping and beating utensils and performing religious rituals' were promulgated (Vysakh and Babu, 2021). These misinformation narratives serve to (temporarily) ease the entropy production associated with fear of the disease, by providing people with alleged, distinct protective measures available within their personal sphere of control. However, that the suggested protective measures are incorrect, and even harmful, meant that over time, entropic production would increase, either through adherents becoming ill with COVID-19 (because they have relied on these measures rather than those based on scientific evidence), or by them succumbing to other diseases related to the proposed 'protections' (such as salmonella infections acquired from cow dung or the Ganga river).

As the pandemic evolved and various restrictive control and mitigation measures were taken by countries, there emerged around the world, a fourth characteristic indicative response, that of *Revolt – You can't control me*. This oppositional attitude constitutes a revolt against the impositions placed upon citizens and usual social and economic interactions, and is grounded in thinking that dismisses the pandemic as not a real threat, as hugely exaggerated or as motivated by conspiratorial agenda.

This attitude is in evidence in the various anti-lockdown, stay-at-home or shelter-in-place protests seen across the world. By mid-April 2020, protests in the US railed against the economic and social impacts of the stay-at-home orders, demanding the re-opening of their respective states, along with a resumption of business and personal activities. In Australia protests escalated with the introduction of repeated, longer and more restrictive 'lock-downs'.

In dismissing the threat of the pandemic as not real or as exaggerated, the protestors demonstrate an anti-governing authority and anti-scientific view, that sees governing authorities as 'liberal elites who are oppressing and corrupting wider society' (MC, 2021). They seek alternative explanations in pandemic 'infodemics' or 'conspiracy theories' as promulgated on social media, that propose 'COVID-19 is a hoax, the vaccine is designed to kill people, or that the recent rollout of 5G technology is to blame for the pandemic' (MC, 2021).

Those in revolt can be interpreted as complex entropic entities whose energetic input does not meet their energetic requirements. Their behaviour indicates they are experiencing significant increase in entropy as high stress. Their 'groan' of suffering, according to those protesting, is linked to loss of income and threat to self-identity through social restrictions. Finding meaning in like-minded community, and not having to expend energy making sense of uncertain futures tend towards requiring less energy and thus, lower entropy production. However, when those in revolt choose an aggressive mode of expression of pain, this is not conducive to generating a sympathetic response across other sectors of society. Disruptive activities, such as protest marches, exacerbate increased levels of entropy across communities. The suffering of disease is potentially increased through exacerbation of situations that foster increased spread of SARS-CoV-2 pathogens. With more people infected, there is greater stress on healthcare systems. Epidemiological studies may then indicate the need for longer and stricter mitigation and control measures, and so increase in potential loss to income and social interactions.

The reactionary formation of conspiracy or denial explanations for dramatic and harmful population-level disasters is an age-old response. Whilst many spiritual, psychological and social theories propose explanations for this style of response, Friston's free energy principle and unified brain theory, outlined in Chapter 2, provides a more fundamental solution to the question of why such thinking evolves. According to Friston, our brains are organised in complex hierarchical layers that act as 'inference generators', perpetually responding to systemic sensory inputs and assessing these against predictive schema, with the goal being to minimise the differences between 'sensation' and 'representation' to minimise entropy (Friston, 2010). Hence, the need for agreement between the interiority and exteriority of our experience emerges from the tendencies of the structure of relations of our bodily-psychological whole-parts and social organisation, to find a steady state of lowest entropy production, often between dialectical or opposing extrema.

Faced with evidence from their sensory phenomena, signalling suffering, against an exteriority of worsening structural disintegration, people turned to new explanatory models that altered the meaning-making of their suffering and reduced cognitive dissonance between that which they felt and observed, and what the causal relationship between those experiences was purported to be by external agencies.

'Revolt', we argue, is the underlying position from which action was taken to seek relief from suffering amongst conspiracy and denialist theorists. Some individuals, organisations, and even governments have taken a hostile and aggressive opposition to both the realities of the pandemic and the mechanisms used by governments to impose restrictions on the reproduction rate of the viral infection, that in turn impose alternative sources of suffering.

Counterposing this extreme is an alternative stance of radical acceptance of the inevitability of overwhelming pandemic infection rates such that 'nature should take its course', with perhaps some limited preventative strategies around vulnerable people. In both positions, cognitive dissonance and the need to expend energy on processing new ways of thinking are effectively rendered inert, because, according to the logic of these positions, either (1) there is no pandemic/it's a conspiracy by powerful people over which I have no control/it's just the flu or (2) nothing can stop the spread/only herd immunity can save us/survival of the fittest.

The specific content of either extreme is less important than the degree of radicalisation. The language of the positions at the extremes also provides clues to other entropic reasons for these radical positions. Conspiracy content often invoke the analogy that people who follow the mainstream current of ideas are acting as 'lambs', as essentially incapable of independent thought or action and critical reasoning. Many advocating for radical acceptance, characterised adherents to ideas about 'flattening the curve' and mitigating social, economic, and health harms through government restrictions, as leftist ideologues who were using the pandemic as an opportunity for radical political change. In each position, the humanity of those in disagreement with the radical perspective has been diminished, and by doing this, the ethical knot of self-other responsibility is loosened.

Suffering triggered radicalisation, as impacts on the structures of society, and the interdependencies upon which people relied for the energetic resources necessary to resist entropic decay continued, despite individual and collective efforts. The development of opposing extrema is an inevitable emergent phenomenon in complex social relations, because of underlying biological, social, and cognitive predispositions that seek to make meaning by harmonising the interiority and exteriority of human experience. Emergent polarities provide a new dialectic within which social order can re-organise and allows for the discharge of the tensions that drive entropic increase. Creating an 'us and them' mentality relieves ethical uncertainty and loosens the knot of responsibility, such that one's future actions or inactions can no longer be interpreted as a violation of self-other responsibility.

Phase 4: Reduced transmission (elimination or eradication measures)

At the time of writing, the SARS-CoV-2 pandemic has not reached this fourth, reduced transmission stage. However, with the development of effective vaccinations, there is now promise that global reduced transmission is possible, providing the vaccines become equitably and widely accessible.

Both elimination (no sustained transmission in a specific region or country), and eradication (no global cases), of COVID-19, remain a challenge. As Michael Osterholm, an epidemiologist at the University of Minnesota, describes it, 'Eradicating this virus right now from the world is a lot like trying to plan the construction of a stepping-stone pathway to the Moon. It's unrealistic' (Phillips, 2021).

According to a Nature survey (Phillips, 2021) of 100 immunologists, infectious disease researchers and virologists working on COVID-19, 89% of respondents envisage that SARS-CoV-2 will continue to be found in particular people or in certain areas into the future.

The arrival of SARS-CoV-2 in a country, with the potential to increase COVID-19 related morbidity and mortality, can be viewed as a perturbation to the homeostatic conditions of a country. This triggers actions by the governing authorities, to reduce disease transmission by mitigating the spread (social isolation measures) and attending to preparedness strategies (increasing medical research, hospital capacity) while also seeking to re-assure citizens, and mitigate detrimental effects on the economy and habits of daily life.

While research into the development of a vaccine was being undertaken, the mitigation and control measures available comprised integrated non-pharmacological interventions: Rigorous surveillance, early detection and isolation of cases and limitation to pathways via which the pathogen might transmit between humans. Some countries performed better in securing the necessary infrastructure and modifying individual and organisational behaviours to suppress viral reproduction.

The Lowy Institute, in exploring how more than 100 countries managed reduction in disease transmission in the 43 weeks following their 100th COVID-19 case (using data available to 13 March 2021), found that a complex picture emerged of evolving strategies, time frames of successful strategy implementation, and social compliance. For example, structural factors, such as a smaller population, cohesive societies and effective organisations, had some advantage in dealing with the pandemic; developing countries were more successful in mitigating the initial outbreak; countries with higher average *per capita* wealth performed better as the pandemic continued; and, the wealth of the country was associated with better access to vaccines and hence population immunity and positive outcomes.

Haug et al. (2020), in assessing the effectiveness of over 6,000 non-pharmaceutical interventions (NPIs), implemented across 79 jurisdictions, found that social distancing and movement restriction measures, such as curfews, lockdowns, work at home orders, travel restrictions, border closures, and closures of places where people gather in small groups (shops, schools and so on) were the most effective NPIs. However, they also note that these measures cause the most disruption to societies, economic activities and human rights.

In sum, drawing on the factors as indicated by the Lowy Institute and Huang et al., and reflecting on the characteristic response attitudes as discussed above, we conclude that the success of social mitigation responses is: Dependent on social and government trust and interconnectedness; time-dependent; varied over time based on how the population responded to and sustained efforts; contingent on initial conditions; and requiring a series of interconnected mechanisms and adaptive responses for successful suppression of viral reproduction rates.

However, the most powerful mitigation intervention has been the large-scale vaccination roll-outs, beginning towards the end of 2020. Vaccination is a profoundly anti-entropic mechanism. In the first instance, as a non-random injection of energy, vaccination penetrates deep and wide into the stratum of the complex whole-part of the human host reservoir. Despite a small effect individually, it has the potential to suppress infection reproduction rates and dramatically reduce the burden of infection amongst populations. Such an effect has been key to the promise of a normalisation of personal and collective ways of interacting. Promisingly, despite viral adaptations and evolution within host systems, early evidence from whole-of-population vaccination programs shows they have been effective at limiting the viral spread and reducing the burden on health services around the world (Henry et al., 2021).

The interdependency between virus, host, and populations means that the mechanism of induced non-pathogenic immunity, dramatically resolves a key driver of the entropic increase manifested by the pandemic. Immunity confers highly significant information across an enormous set of critical interdependencies, revolving around viral hosts and their contact with others in the potential host reservoir. As a result, the population restrictions to contain viral reproduction become less critical as the rate of reproduction, and the consequences of infection, are moderated by vaccine-induced immunity.

However, with the evolution of new variants, such as Delta and Omicron, vaccination regimes have had to be revised to provide necessary population immunity. Prior to global access to, and implementation of, effective vaccine regimes against new variants, control measures of rigorous surveillance, early detection and isolation of cases continue to be necessary to reduce disease transmission.

More than two years into the presence of SARS-CoV-2, the characteristic indicative responses to evidence of a viral pandemic and associated restrictive and control measures, as previously discussed, continue to be at play in social and government responses. Attitudinal responses of dismissal, complacency and revolt are evidenced in an article in the Australian newspaper, Daily Telegraph (MacDonald, 2021). Journalist Heather MacDonald, in her piece 'Peddling fear not facts', argues that the Australian government measures to mitigate the spread of the Omicron variant serve as a case study 'in the deliberate manufacture of fear' (ibid., p. 13). She cites as a key strategy in the manufacture of fear, that the 'officials' 'buttress group fear with expert opinion'. One of the experts that she claims is determined to 'put the most dire spin on Omicron' is the Director General of the WHO, Dr. Tedros Adhanom Ghbreyesus, who she quotes as saying 'Even if Omicron causes less severe cases, the sheer number of cases could once again overwhelm unprepared health systems' (ibid., p. 13). MacDonald proposes that 'There are apparently no circumstances that would warrant a less-than-totalitarian response in advance of any actual disaster' (ibid., p. 13). For those who respect the expert medical opinion of the world's peak healthcare organisation and its Director General, MacDonald's argument is incomprehensible. However, MacDonald's sentiments are a reminder that throughout all phases of the pandemic, the views of sectors of society who do not value or understand scientific and medical knowledge and evidence, will continue to exert influence.

Summative discussion of government and societal responses to SARS-CoV-2

The survey of government and societal responses to SARS-CoV-2 illustrates how phrase space shapes the habits of thought of individuals (governing authority figures, citizens) and the taken for granted assumptions of various collectives (governments, social sectors), and exerts self-imposed limitations on sense making preferences.

In the four indicative characteristic attitudes to the pandemic, we see how the phrase space and communicative connectedness of people shaped responses. Citizens and governing authorities with little experience and understanding of scientific and medical knowledge were not always convinced by these modes of explanation nor for the need for certain measures to be taken to mitigate the effects of the virus. On the other hand, those who identified with these discourses or phrase spaces or those who had trust in medical experts (communicative connectedness), took the advice.

Across countries, governing authorities, societies and individuals, there is evidence of significant entropic increase with the spread of the pandemic. In societies in which there were lower levels of pre-existing expectation and readiness for a pandemic, decisions had to be made in situations of relatively high uncertainty (high informational entropy) for the expenditure of vast economic, social, and emotional resources. Whether the starting point was one predominated by dismissal or complacency, as the pandemic evolved, the interconnectedness of agents and the coordination of mechanisms to respond to the threat of the pandemic informed the success of how those resources were expended.

With news, then arrival of the COVID-19 pandemic, individuals and collectives expended energy in interpreting evidence of its severity and learning about preparedness, control and mitigation strategies. Energy for a range of other responsibilities and tasks became unavailable as governing authorities instituted necessary containment and mitigation measures, and societies and citizens learned how to manage new daily patterns of life.

Uncertainty increased as governing authorities grappled with understanding the necessary and most effective types and timing of interventions to minimise incidence, morbidity and mortality, while also minimising disruptions to economic, political and social activities. In the context of unprecedented restrictions, there was a noticeable increase in felt uncertainty about what the daily rhythms, increased physical isolation and loss of income would mean in social, political and economic terms. Whereas prior to the pandemic, for many people, their sense of self and patterns of living were taken for granted and established, the restrictions associated with managing the pandemic meant the question 'How then shall we live?' became overt and urgent.

Increased incidence of depression and anxiety disorders associated with the pandemic attests to the profound entropic impact of the pandemic on the interiority and exteriority of people's lived experience. The material, emotional and cognitive costs to individuals and societies were substantial and forced a re-organisation or re-set of people's prior states.

Entropic increase due to information loss was in evidence across governments, societies and in individuals. For example, although the WHO had predicted a new pandemic would occur at some time, advocated country and global preparedness, understood the expected phases of development and most effective management strategies, many governing authorities appeared not to have assimilated this information. Rather, it appeared that governing authorities, societies, organisations and individuals learnt their way through the pandemic. With complex self-organising entities such as people, societies, organisations and governments, 'information' generated by others, becomes part of the environment within which they exist and dynamically interact. Complex entities choose what they notice and how they respond. So, information generated by WHO does not equate with information engaged with by the authorities tasked with managing responses to SARS-CoV-2. Similarly, there is loss of information and consequent increase in entropy evident as individuals and community groups are informed about the severity and contagiousness of COVID-19. Self-organising sense-making of this information means that while some believe the validity of the information, and react with concern, others seek alternative misinformation or simply do not understand the importance of physical distancing measures to halt viral spread.

It is evident that the ethical knot of self-other responsibility to relieve or avoid suffering, whether informed by authoritarian or liberal political persuasions, remained a central attractor around which actions emerged. Governments sought to protect their citizens from SARS-CoV-2, to be prepared to care for those who did become sick and to limit the social and economic pain inflicted by whole-of-population relational disruptions caused by the essential re-organisation of the structure of relations of society.

The functioning of healthcare organisations in the midst of a pandemic

The preceding survey illustrates how government and social responses to the COVID-19 pandemic arise through socially interacting agents (citizens, medical experts, governing authorities). These interactions between agents can be understood as entropic exchanges and transformations that vary according to how the strategic responses of each country unfold. The responses of healthcare organisations likewise emerge through socially interacting agents and are reliant upon multiple interdependencies. These interactions too, are traceable through study of entropic flow.

COVID-19 has enormously affected healthcare organisations (hospitals, private clinics, medical research laboratories, health promotion and research institutions and so on) worldwide. Preparations for potential major outbreaks, together with changes to policies and routine practices to protect patients and the healthcare workforce from contamination, while treating infected and non-COVID-19 patients, means individuals and collectives have had to quickly adapt to situations as they evolve.

With the healthcare arrangements of a country dynamically entwined with the history of social and government preferences, per capita wealth, population size, along with regional and global relationships, the functioning of healthcare organisations in the midst of a pandemic reflect these multiple local, regional and global interdependencies. This means that mechanisms for preventing, detecting and responding to the outbreak of a pandemic, emerge reciprocally through the governing authorities, society and healthcare organisations of a country, in the context of global interconnections.

To quickly adapt to emerging circumstances, individuals and collectives require the ability to make informed adaptive responses. To be informed, people need to be in effective communicative relationships with appropriate and knowledgeable others. To be adaptive, there needs to be a culture of democratic individuality in healthcare organisations, that allows individuals discernment and choice within boundaries.

Clay-Williams, Rapport and Braithwaite (2020) describe the ability of a healthcare organisation to 'adjust its functioning prior to, during, or following events (changes, disturbances, and opportunities), and thereby sustain required operations under both expected and unexpected conditions' (ibid., p. 1) as resilience. In the language of complexity, resilience signifies the ability to freely make informed adaptive responses.

The demands of a pandemic propel healthcare organisations to adjust functioning, while sustaining required operations, under emerging crisis conditions. Resilience is thus critical for healthcare organisations to adequately respond to the evolving dynamics of the COVID-19 crisis. Resilience is tied to communicative connectedness: Levels of trust and coherence between agents. Strong communicative connectedness amongst multiple interdependencies (such as governing authorities, medical practitioners, manufacturers of medical supplies, local healthcare agencies and so on), is necessary for organisations to adjust functioning with minimal energetic input.

Interactions between these various agents implicate entropic exchanges. With multiple interacting agents dynamically responding to one another, and learning their way through to how to sustain required operations, strong communicative connectedness between agents is necessary to limit entropic increase and thereby enable more agile whole of healthcare responses during a pandemic.

Thus, resilience is reliant on strong communicative connectedness between the dynamically interacting entropic agents, whereby entropy development within, and across agents and organisations, is minimised. In this way, resilience supports the capacity of healthcare practitioners to provide high quality care to suffering patients. Further, resilience protects healthcare practitioners from experiencing work related sustained stress and thereby becoming vulnerable to the development of illness.

This framing draws attention to how interactions, including those beyond healthcare organisations, shape the capacity of practitioners to minimise the entropic increase of a patient. For example, practitioner stress is exacerbated if a government has not arranged for manufacture of sufficient PPE, and this negatively affects their capacity to provide high quality healthcare (minimisation of entropy in the suffering patient).

Principles for optimising healthcare during a pandemic

We can learn how to optimise healthcare during a pandemic, by examining the experiences of practitioners, and the strategies undertaken by healthcare organisations to cultivate resilience (the minimisation of entropic increase across the organisation).

Research into healthcare practitioners' experiences of working with COVID-19 (Bennett et al., 2020; Clay-Williams, Rapport and Braithwaite, 2020) indicates increase in entropy production associated with unavailable energy, uncertainty, disorder/dispersal and loss of information. These authors report exacerbated stress as pressure on everyday dynamic self-organisation associated with, but not limited to: Fear of contracting the virus or passing it on to family and friends; high workloads and long shifts; changing and inconsistent guidelines; inadequate cognisance of clinicians views by senior managers; lack of training; inadequate PPE; inadequate testing; lack of beds and respiratory equipment; new living arrangements (to protect family members); interpersonal isolation; and periods of quarantine. Psychosocial distress, associated with caring for patients as well as keeping themselves and their families safe, along with the physical requirements of new patterns of living, indicates the imposition of additional energy requirements on practitioners.

Taken together these exacerbations of stress, as 'moral distress' (Murray, Kaufman and Williams, 2021), are connected to issues that impact on the capacity of practitioners to care for patients, themselves and their families. The experience of stress as described by practitioners can be interpreted as generated through a core concern of care for the suffering of others. In this interpretation, distress constitutes a manifestation of an innate predisposition to care, as proposed by Levinas (2003). In our ComEntEth model of healthcare, it is this relationship of care, expressed as commitment to reduce suffering or entropy increase in patients, that functions as the central attractor around which healthcare dynamics unfold. In this framing, strategies and mechanisms that facilitate the capacity of practitioners to care for patients, whilst assisting in minimising the practitioners' own entropic increase, are those that optimise the capacity of healthcare during a pandemic.

In an associated point, it is interesting to note that following the first waves of COVID-19 and associated hospitalisations, practitioners reported experiencing exacerbated distress associated with caring for those people who have refused vaccination and subsequently succumbed to the disease. In circumstances where patients could have protected themselves and others through taking a vaccination, and where they have ended up requiring intensive healthcare interventions, practitioners have reported feeling a sense of moral transgression against themselves (personal communication).

Framed in terms of Levinas's philosophy of an ethics of responsibility, the practitioners are not being treated as being in a relationship of responsibility with the patient. This feeling of not being valued as a human being by the patient adds to the practitioner's stress and thus raises their entropy levels.

There is currently a burgeoning of research into lessons learned during the COVID-19 pandemic about how to facilitate effective functioning of healthcare during a pandemic (see, for example, Clay-Williams, Rapport and Braithwaite, 2020; Murray, Kaufman and Williams, 2021). The principles, strategies and detailed practical actions recommended in this research, describe how resilience is facilitated and, in the terms of our thesis, how stress and entropy production is minimised. In essence, these principles, strategies and detailed practical actions address the means by which the capacity of practitioners to care for the suffering patient can be maximised. For example, through adequate supply of correctly fitting PPE, re-arrangement of beds and equipment to enable easier monitoring of patients or daily cross organisational hub meetings to keep everyone informed of the situation.

Two major themes are apparent in the reflections and recommendations regarding the functioning of healthcare organisations in a pandemic. The first is the importance of communicative connectedness. Researchers describe how a regular means of information sharing, as well as opportunities for the practitioners to have their views considered, was important for managing personal stress and anxiety, and fostering a supportive culture. This refers as much to communication between healthcare institutions and governing authorities, as to between hospitals and other healthcare organisations (such as pathology clinics), sections, teams, clinicians and senior managers.

A complexity perspective emphasises how relationships and communicative connectedness critically shape the unfolding of complex phenomena. The contours of the communicative connectedness sought, align with the major principles of Etienne Wenger's concept of 'communities of practice' (Wenger, 1998), whereby a group of people meet and interact regularly, so as to learn how to improve their shared practice. This is an apt description of the communal learning sought, that allows healthcare organisations to quickly and effectively respond to COVID-19 associated changed circumstances.

The second major theme is the importance of the capacity of healthcare practitioners to make informed, self-organised, dynamic responses to unfolding situations. As Murray, Kaufman and Williams (2021) note, where 'home-grown' interventions are supported, whereby the actors in various healthcare situations create solutions to immediate needs (such as delivering workshops, creating material for websites, developing pathways to facilitate PPE access or re-organising the physical layout), necessary organisational flexibility is made possible.

In sum, democratic individualism in conjunction with strong communicative connectedness' promotes organisational resilience and hence the capacity of the healthcare organisation to swiftly respond to the changing circumstances of the COVID-19 crisis.

Concluding comments

In this chapter, we have demonstrated the utility of studying government, social and organisational responses from the perspective of our ComEntEth model, to make sense of why and how the world has evolved different outcomes in relation to the shared crisis of the COVID-19 pandemic.

Our exposition has foregrounded how through multiple modes of increased entropy production (unavailable energy, disorder/dispersal, uncertainty and information loss), individuals, communities and countries have struggled to make sense of, and coordinate, mechanisms to stem the impact of the pandemic on personal, economic and social structures of relations. What resulted were severe and sustained disruptions to the rhythms of life, the interdependencies of agencies, and the allocation of collective and personal capital. These effects were sensitive to initial conditions. Those countries with recent experience of dealing with a pandemic required less energy to re-organise patterns of behaviour and relating, to successfully moderate the impact of COVID-19.

The importance of preparation and planning, involving all layers of society, from the individual to the collective, to minimise the entropic cost of a pandemic, was highlighted. Uncertainty about appropriate steps to take and consequent rapid re-organising, manifests as entropic rise in individuals and collectives. Preparation and planning can be understood as constituting a collective cognitive offloading strategy, a means of supporting memory for delayed intentions (Boldt and Gilbert, 2019), such as necessary mechanisms to engage when there is a pandemic. Where governing authorities and societal institutions have a means of quickly accessing an intention (preparation and planning for a pandemic), the entropic cost will be lessened.

In the context of easily accessed global communications, any disconnect between public messaging by authorities and the lived experience of people, undermines trust in those authorities and thus communicative connectedness between governing authorities, societies and institutions will be fractured. This then undermines the pandemic response efforts of those in authority and facilitates non-compliance in citizens.

Management of a pandemic requires a whole of society response, and for an effective whole of society response to a pandemic, there needs to be strong communicative connectedness between governing authorities, societies and healthcare organisations. Through communicative connectedness greater shared understanding can evolve which assists in minimising individual and collective entropic rise. Entropy production is minimised where there is a stronger sense of certainty about what needs to be done, effective information communication and less energy expended in stress. This supports more efficient efforts to control and mitigate the spread of a pandemic so that entropic rise associated with disease is likewise minimised.

References

Bennett, P., Noble, S., Johnston, S., Jones, D. and Hunter, R. (2020) 'COVID-19 Confessions: A Qualitative Exploration of Healthcare Workers Experiences of Woking with COVID-19'. *British Medical Journal Open*. 10:e043949.

Bergquist, S., Otten, T. and Sarich, N. (2020) 'COVID-19 Pandemic in the United States'. *Health Policy Technology*. 9(4):623–638.

Boldt, A. and Gilbert, S. J. (2019) 'Confidence Guides Spontaneous Cognitive Offloading'. *Cognitive Research: Principles and Implications*. 4:45.

Centers for Disease Control and Prevention (2021) *COVID Data Tracker*. Covid. cdc.gov.

Chan, S. (July 27, 2020) *Leading Hong Kong's Response to Coronavirus*. Boston: Harvard T. H. Chan School of Public Health.

Claeson, M. and Hanson, S. (2020) 'COVID-19 and the Swedish Enigma'. *The Lancet*. 397(10271):259–261.

Clay-Williams, R., Rapport, F. and Braithwaite, J. (2020) 'The Australian Health System Response to COVID-19 from a Resilient Health Care Perspective: What Have We Learned?' *Public Health Research and Practice*. 30(4):e3042025.

Coveney, P. and Highfield, R. (1996) *Frontiers of Complexity*. London: Faber and Faber.

Friston, K. (2010) 'The Free Energy Principle: A Unified Brain Theory?'. *Nature Reviews*. 11:126–137.

Haug, N., Geyrhofer, L., Londei, A., Dervic, E., DesvarLarrive, A., Loreto, V., Pinior, B., Thurner, S. and Klimek, P. (2020) 'Ranking the Effectiveness of Worldwide COVID-19 Government Interventions'. *Nature Human Behaviour*. 4:1303–1312.

Henry, D., Jones, M. Stehlik, P. and Glassziou, P. (2021) 'Effectiveness of COVID-19 Vaccines: Findings from Real World Studies'. *The Medical Journal of Australia* [Preprint, 20 May 2021].

Hidayat, S. E., Farooq, M. O. and Alim, E. A. (Eds) (2020) *The Impact of the COVID-19 Outbreak on Islamic Finance in the OIC Countries*. Komite Nasional Ekonomi dan Keuangan Syariah National (KNEKS) (National Committee for Islamic Economy and Finance): Indonesia.

Kuhn, L. (2009) *Adventures in Complexity for Organisations Near the Edge of Chaos*. Axminster: Triarchy Press.

Levinas, E. (2003) 'Useless Suffering'. Bernasconi, R. and Wood, D. (Eds) *The Provocation of Levinas: Rethinking the Other* (R. Cohen, Trans). London: Routledge.

Lowy Institute (2021) *Covid Performance Index*. https://interactives.lowyinstitute.org/features/covid-performance/

MacDonald, H. (Dec. 24, 2021) 'Peddling Fear, Not Facts'. Surrey Hills, NSW, Australia. *Daily Telegraph.*

Martin, S. (Sept. 8, 2021) 'Pfizer Asked to Meet With Greg Hunt About "Millions of Doses" of Vaccine But Was Offered Bureaucrat Instead'. *The Guardian.* australia@theguardian.com

MC, A. (Oct. 5, 2021) 'Australia's Far Right Gets COVID Anti-Lockdown Protest Booster'. *Al Jazeera.*www.aljazeera.com

Morens, D. M., Folkers, G.K. and Fauci, A. S. (2009) 'What Is a Pandemic?'. *The Journal of Infectious Diseases.* 200(7):1018–1021.

Morin, E. (2008) *On Complexity* (R. Postel and M. Kelly, Trans). NJ: Hampton Press.

Murray, E., Kaufman, K. R. and Williams, R. (2021) 'Let Us Do Better: Learning Lessons for Recovery of Healthcare Professionals During and After COVID-19'. *BJPsych Open.* 7(5):E151. doi:10.1192/bjo.2021.981

Phillips, N. (Feb. 16, 2021) 'The Coronavirus Is Here to Stay: Here's What That Means'. *Nature.* 590:382–384.

Prigogine, I. (1980) *From Being to Becoming: Time and Complexity in the Physical Sciences.* San Francisco: Freeman.

Ranney, M., Griffeth, V. and Jha, A. (2020) 'Critical Supply Shortages: The Need for Ventilators and Personal Protective Equipment During the Covid-19 Pandemic'. *New England Medicine.* 382:e41.

Saiidi, U. (July 2, 2020) 'How Hong Kong Beat Coronavirus and Avoided Lockdown'. *CNBC.*

Santomauro, D. (2021) 'Global Prevalence and Burden of Depressive and Anxiety Disorders in 204 Countries and Territories in 2020 Due to the COVID-19 Pandemic'. *The Lancet.* 398(10312):1700–1712.

Seale, H., Heywood, A. E., Leask, J., Sheel, M., Thomas, S., Durrheim, D. N., Bolsewicz, K. and Kaur, R. (2020) 'COVID-19 Is Rapidly Changing: Examining Public Perceptions and Behaviours in Response to This Evolving Pandemic'. *PLOS One.* 15(6):e0235112.

Tsirtsakis, A. (2020) 'Australians, COVID-19 and the question of complacency.'racgp. org.au/newsgp/clinical/social-responsibility-vs-adherence-to-the-rules-covid

Viglione, G. (Sept. 3, 2020) 'Four Ways Trump Has Meddled in Pandemic Sciences: Why It Matters'. *Nature Human Behaviour.*www.nature.com/articles/d41586-020-03035-4

Vysakh, C. and Babu, R. H. (Mar. 2021) 'COVID-19 Infodemic and Misinfodemic: A Tale of India'. *Academic Letters.* Article 799.

Wenger, E. (1998) *Communities of Practice.* Cambridge: Cambridge University Press.

World Health Organization (2018) *Managing Epidemics: Key Facts About Major Deadly Diseases.* Geneva: World Health Organization.

World Health Organization (2020a) *Report of the WHO-China Joint Mission on Coronavirus Disease 2019 (COVID-19).* Geneva: World Health Organization.

World Health Organization (2020b) *WHO: Timeline – COVID-19.* Geneva: World Health Organization.

Zerofsky, E. (Apr. 9, 2020) 'How Viktor Orban Used the Coronavirus to Seize More Power'. *The New Yorker.*

5 Afterword

Complexity, Entropy and Ethics in Healthcare

Introduction

Somewhere between the senselessness of perfect order and the meaningless-ness of perfect chaos, life takes hold. Within the infinitely complex bound-aries of these extrema, the mechanisms, structures and physical energies driving the functions of life on earth arise within a narrow band of transac-tions and transformations of matter and potential energies that, on the scale of the universal, approach an equilibrium of absolute zero. Approach, but fundamentally never reach it, always existing in a non-equilibrium flux of forces and flows between matter, free energy, and entropy. This relatively tiny set of boundaries, which in our book we define as homeostasis, pro-vides exactly the necessary distance from equilibrium to allow for the cou-pling and dissipation of physical properties of the matter and energy of the systems of life to resist, and even thrive on, the inevitable energetic march towards maximum entropy.

As French philosopher Edgar Morin reminds us, 'It is this dialogic of order and disorder that produces all of the living organisations in the uni-verse' (Morin, 2008, p. 87) and as such, people exist as a mixture of order and disorder, maintained by homeostatic processes around entropic flows.

These considerations have informed our articulation of a secure philo-sophical grounding for healthcare. In seeking a deeper understanding of 'what is really going on' in the practice of healthcare, we have found in the complexity sciences, studies of entropy in living organisms, and the ethics of Emmanuel Levinas, a satisfying means of conceptualising the structure of relations in healthcare. Our theorising of healthcare as complex, entropic and ethical, resolved in our ComEntEth (Complex Entropic Ethical) model which addresses underlying ontological, epistemological and axiological assumptions.

By a 'secure philosophical grounding for healthcare', we mean an explana-tion that has philosophical coherence and practical utility. We describe our

DOI: 10.4324/9781003197454-5

undertaking as applied philosophy, because it is concerned with highly abstract principles addressing beliefs about ontology (What kind of being is a human? What is the nature of reality?), epistemology (the nature of knowledge) and axiology (values and ethics), and the implications of these for practice.

As complex thinking positions the human observer as participating in a relational universe – we are part of that upon which we philosophically reflect – our theorising begins from a place of epistemological uncertainty and humility. So, in developing a secure philosophical grounding for health-care, we do so with this awareness. Our stance could be described as co-constructivist (Kuhn, 2009; Morin, 2008) whereby we recognise that 'we construct our perception of the world, but with the help of the world itself which, as it were, lends us a hand' (Morin, 2008, p. 91), or critical realism (Fleetwood, 2004; Le Plastrier, 2019) that similarly recognises contingency and partial indeterminacy in human knowing.

In this chapter, we summarise the central thesis and main themes of the book and reflect on the implications of our ComEntEth theoretical framing for improving management of the complexity of healthcare.

Central thesis and main themes

The theorising in this book comprises an approach to studying how people get things done in organisations, specifically in healthcare organisations. As such, it is concerned with sense making in the social sciences, and one of the sites of interest within this, organisation studies. So, although we have drawn on findings and ideas from the complexity sciences, thermodynamics and bio-medicine, we have translated and interpreted these from the perspective of human social and organisational activity. In so doing, we have made links between complexity concepts, the second law of thermodynamics, and ethical thinking, to generate new ways to conceptualise the mechanisms and relations through which the behaviour of individuals, departments, institutions and sectors arise.

We were provoked into writing this book because of our sense that despite the substantial body of research into interactions between patients, practitioners and managers, there was a lack of a global integrated and explicit discourse around the ontological, epistemological and axiological framing of healthcare.

In our opinion, cognisance of a coherent theoretical framing of the structure of relations in healthcare, that addresses ontological, epistemological and axiological precepts, is an essential beginning point to consideration of how healthcare may be improved. Often improvements are targeted at changing practice in order to achieve certain pre-determined outcomes (such as reducing overcrowding and access blockages in EDs), and often new strategies carry with them unexpected and serious consequences, that at times, might have been avoided had the structure of relations in healthcare been better understood.

The structure of relations we propose, is as stated in our fundamental postulate: *That in **complex** phenomena, such as healthcare, complexity unfolds in **entropic** flows, under the influence of an **ethical** attractor.* We have named this conceptualisation the ComEntEth model of healthcare. Specifically, we theorise that the central attractor revealed through the self-organising activities of those involved in healthcare, is the desire to reduce elevated entropy or suffering in patients, with this occurring through ethically motivated energetic interventions from practitioner to patient.

As the complexity sciences are concerned with study into how multiple interacting and evolving systems (from the cellular to the social) give rise to emergent collective behaviours, they constitute an appropriate approach to illuminating the complexity of healthcare.

Characterising the multiple interactions by which healthcare is manifest, as energetic transactions and transformations whereby entropic production is managed, provides further information about how emergent collective behaviours arise. Levinas's ethics of self-other responsibility corresponds with the complexity sciences relational view of human beings, and extends the thermodynamic explanation of the power of energetic interventions to reduce the entropic increase of suffering as trauma and disease. In both a thermodynamic and ethical sense, the groan of suffering can be understood to elicit a response from others to alleviate suffering. From Levinas's perspective, we are ethically motivated to reduce suffering in the other, because their suffering elicits in us, recognition of our own suffering.

In conceptualising healthcare as complex, entropic and ethical, we propose that:

- Healthcare is constituted by energetic relational exchanges between people, as self-organising, dynamic and emergent entities.
- These energetic relational exchanges unfold around a central attractor, reduction in suffering or entropy production in patients, through the healthcare practitioner offering appropriate energetic interventions.
- This process is made possible through humans being in a relationship of responsibility and care for one another.

The logic of our ComEntEth conceptualisation of healthcare, as outlined in this book, is that:

- Humans, as complex entities, manage internal entropy (health and wellness) through homeostatic processes.

- Suffering constitutes a phenomenological experience of entropic over-whelm of homeostatic processes (trauma and disease).
- When the causal relations and mechanisms of internal homeostasis are overwhelmed, the suffering person (patient) turns outwards for assistance.
- Healthcare practitioners seek to ameliorate suffering (elevated entropy) by offering interventions to reduce entropy production in the patient.
- This interaction between patient and healthcare practitioner is central to the capacity of healthcare to reduce entropy production.
- The *raison d'etre* across all activities in healthcare is the principle of seeking to reduce elevated entropy production.
- Minimisation of entropy production in healthcare practitioners and across the multiple relationships constituting healthcare, supports the capacity of practitioners to reduce the patient's elevated entropy.

Implications for practice

Our ComEntEth model presents a conception of healthcare where, no matter the scale of focus, global system, sector, organisation, department or the individuals involved, complexity in healthcare is viewed as arising through myriad entropic transactions and transformations that cohere around efforts to reduce suffering or entropic levels in patients.

The value of viewing healthcare from the novel ComEntEth model, outlined in this book, lies with the potential for gaining beneficial new insights that lead to improvement in practice.

One new insight is that, by viewing the processes and practices of healthcare as energetic transactions and transformations or entropic flow, we can identify the dynamic capacity, character of interactions and longevity of healthcare organisations, be they departments, clinics, sectors and so on. Viewing each functional unit of healthcare as entropic, we can examine how the energetic input meets or fails to meet, the energetic requirements of the entity. Evidence of the energetic requirements not being met will be displayed as increased entropy production in the organisational unit and individual practitioners involved (as increased stress and distress), and ineffective practices that may endanger patient health, rather than ameliorate suffering. Therefore, awareness of entropic production across healthcare is important, as this provides information about the adaptive 'self-eco-organising' of the people and organisations involved, as well as indications of how entropic flow, and thus healthcare, might be improved

A second major new insight is that our ComEntEth model fosters an integral perspective that encompasses biological, social and psychological aspects of healthcare. This perspective highlights how entropic flow unifies fundamental energetic material evolution over time, in biological and sociological structures of relations, within individual people and the social organisations they create. Explaining complex interactions in healthcare as entropic transactions presents a unified way of perceiving trauma and illness, their alleviating treatments, and the myriad complex relationships manifest in healthcare. In particular, how bio-medicine and organisational dynamics are conjoined in efforts to manage the elevated entropy or suffering of patients is highlighted.

In the following, we identify some of the crucial benefits of theorising healthcare in terms of each of the three domains of our model.

Benefits of theorising complexity in healthcare organisations

Making sense of the complexity of healthcare through consideration of the self-eco-organising of the individuals, organisations, populations and environments involved, builds insight into new ways to conceive, and construct, solutions to improve the practice of healthcare.

Freed from the bonds of linear, reductionist assumptions, the messiness and uncertainty described and lived by patients, healthcare workers, administrators, and health bureaucrats are no longer 'latent variables' to be 'controlled for', but instead assume their proper place as inevitabilities of the world in which healthcare unfolds. Messiness, uncertainty and the paradoxical character of situations produced through everyday relational exchanges are understood to be features of complexity that imbue healthcare with the capacity to change and evolve over time.

A complexity view highlights the intimate relationship between the individual actions of those involved and healthcare manifestation at any point in time. The notion of causality, as linear and directed, can be re-conceptualised as both latent and emergent properties of particular, and often myriad, self-organising and dynamic interactions between all involved in the particular site of practice.

A complexity perspective reminds us of how the efficacy of the words and deeds of one individual cannot be determined in isolation, nor in advance, but rather evolves through interaction and cooperation with other self-organising, dynamic and emerging people. This is because individual undertakings, including speech, being inserted into a network of relationships between self-eco-organising people, each with their own centres of initiative (thoughts, feelings and actions), sets in train unpredictable and often irreversible responses (Dunne, 1993).

A complexity view of how organisational behaviours emerge, recognises that:

> Widespread patterns of behaviour are always implicated in individual
> action, which means that individual action and the actions of groups,

organisations or societies cannot be seen as something happening at different levels. Rather, actions are contributing to different scales of behaviour.

(Johannessen and Kuhn, 2012, p. xi)

Structures of organisation can be understood to emerge over time, through dynamic interactions between self-organising human beings. Poet Phillip Larkin (1988) in his poem 'The daily things we do' evokes this understanding of how, through the 'doing' of individual agents over time, organisational behaviour, culture and structure, emerges: 'The circumstances we cause/In time gives rise to us/Becomes our memory'.

Two important points are useful to consider when thinking about emergence in healthcare. The first is to recognise that unexpected behaviours arise through multiple interactions. The second is to be mindful of how micro-phenomena gives rise to macro-phenomena. For example, the well-being of individual practitioners can colour the character and effectiveness of whole departments.

A complexity perspective reminds us that healthcare sectors and organisations do not have to be organised in a pre-ordained way, and show us how organisational structures, or patterns of behaviour, evolve over time as an outcome of the intentions, thinking, feeling and doing of the people involved. These evolved structures then moderate the dynamic self-eco-organising interactions and emergence of those involved. In taking this view, we recognise how both agency and structure are reciprocally implicated in shaping organisation culture and norms of behaviour. This view also explains how both change and constancy are created through multiple interactions, rather than in a top down fashion via imposed directives.

Complexity habits of thought, metaphors and vocabularies not only foster awareness of how the processes and practices of healthcare emerge out of complex self-eco-organisation, but offer ways to identify pattern and potentiality that are not tied to linear and reductionist assumptions:

- *Phase/phrase space*, helps identify how various departments, institutions and sectors generate their own specific organisational dynamics (cultures and behaviours).
- *Communicative connectedness* provides information about the nature and quality of relationships and so can show why certain problems arise and how entropic flow can be improved.
- *Sensitive dependence on initial conditions* reminds us to take the circumstances of concern as a starting point and then track back into the history of the situation to learn why things have emerged in the way they have.
- *Attractors* help managers to constructively review work practices and identify the major forces driving and sustaining behaviours.

- *Fractality* means recognising that as the global and local are embedded in all levels of healthcare practice, whatever the focus of our investigation, there will be information about other levels of the organisation.

Benefits of theorising entropy in healthcare organisations

Theorising entropy in healthcare is beneficial because it directs attention to the fundamental principle whereby life exists. No matter the health system ensemble, cell, bodily organ, patient, practitioner or healthcare sector, attention to entropic exchanges provides a way of making better sense of why certain outcomes are more or less likely, and showing where energetic interventions are necessary to improve health outcomes.

Thinking in terms of 'entropy' provides a way to interrogate, and extend, understanding of the complex, multi-layered and integral biological and social interactions and adaptations that permeate and cohere clinical, management, administration and policy interactions in healthcare.

Theorising the importance of minimising energetic expenditure across healthcare, to support minimisation of entropy production in the practitioner, so that they are in the best position to deal with the patient's elevated entropy, provides a new and unified way of thinking about healthcare. This perspective directs attention to mindfulness of the effects of entropic reverberations across biological, personal, interpersonal and healthcare organisational spheres.

With the focus of healthcare being provision of care for the patient, this has often meant far less attention is paid to the healthcare practitioner. Practitioner stress and distress though is well recognised as detrimental for the individual, the collective within which they work, and to the quality of care. Consideration of the whole of healthcare in terms of management of entropy means recognising that effective strategies to improve healthcare are those that do not increase entropy production in practitioners.

Entropic indicators, as introduced in Chapter 3, provide evidence of the expression of entropy or stress in organisations, and can be analysed to gain understanding about how to improve the management of complexity in healthcare. Indications of unavailable energy, uncertainty, disorder/dispersal and information loss are useful in providing specific information about what is causing stress/distress and tension in practitioners, and thus direct towards appropriate responses.

Benefits of theorising Levinas's ethics in healthcare organisations

Levinas's ethics of responsibility theorises healthcare as predicated on the relationship between the person who suffers, and the 'other' who provides succour. This framing necessarily construes a structure of relations that is ethically defined.

Theorising healthcare as grounded in Levinas's ethics of responsibility explains the energetic power of suffering. In Levinas's framing, suffering elicits a desire in others to help the suffering person, because of the innate sense of self-other responsibility. This framing unites an ethical and biological explanation of the power of suffering. A biological thermodynamic explanation shows how management of entropy is critical to sustaining the function of cells, organs, individuals, and healthcare organisations. The ethics of self-other responsibility explains the willingness of people to seek to reduce the suffering of others and thereby assist in reducing entropic increase in the person who is suffering. Self-other responsibility based on this framing, can be theorised as both underpinning and activating the existence of healthcare activities in human societies, and unifying an iterative and contingent structure of relations in healthcare, that is organised in response to the universality of entropic flow.

From the perspective of an ethics of responsibility, human existence and a sense of subjectivity are understood to arise from a relationship with, and responsibility for, others. A sense of self-other responsibility provides an explanation for why the increase in entropy production, expressed as suffering, activates others to care for the suffering person. When another person expresses pain or suffering, in empathising with them, in feeling this too could be our pain, we feel a desire to ease their pain. Healthcare as a societal institution can thus be understood to constitute a stylised and formalised means of responding to the suffering of others.

How engaging with the ComEntEth model can foster insights

It seems apposite at this juncture in our summary and reflection to present an example of how engaging with the ComEntEth model can foster improvement in practice.

The scenario 'Caring for Marion', is focused around a single patient history, and was created out of an agglomeration of voices. The clinicians involved were invited to consider their experiences from the perspective of applied ComEntEth principles, and following the scenario, we present their conclusions.

Caring for Marion

Marion presented to a hospital ED with vomiting and epigastric pain that had developed over six hours and on arrival, she was reporting a pain score of 10 out of 10 (10/10). Aged 68, the differential list of possible acute serious or life-threatening pathologies was significant, including gastroenteritis, acute cholecystitis, peptic ulcer disease, pancreatitis, small bowel obstruction, acute myocardial infarct, and dissecting aneurysm. Within ten minutes, she was assessed by the nursing team, given a high priority and reviewed by a physician, and several treatments were initiated.

At this stage, the history did not significantly exclude any of the serious diagnoses, so the treating team commenced parallel treatment protocols, including the acute coronary syndrome pathway, treatment for peptic ulcer and acute pancreatitis, and general opioid-based analgesia. Over the course of an hour, her work up suggested that it was not a heart attack, and physical examination suggested a new painful lump at the site of an old abdominal wall hernia. The treating team's working diagnosis was now an acute bowel obstruction secondary to an incarcerated hernia of the abdominal wall.

The hospital that Marion was being treated in did not have surgical services. She would have to be transferred to another hospital for further surgical management. Prior to transfer her treatment revolved around comfort measures and monitoring vitals to ensure her clinical picture was not deteriorating.

On this particular day, the ED was very busy, with low staff numbers. The nurses were all agency staff who did not usually work in the hospital but were helping out due to staff shortages. The treating physician was personally responsible for the care of 20 patients during their shift but had only slept three hours the night before after being called in to assist with a life-threatening emergency. A phone call to ambulance transport services confirmed that due to very high demand in the community, it would be a couple of hours before they could assist in transferring Marion to a surgical hospital.

Marion's pain was very difficult to control. She continued intermittently to vomit, and her pain score ranged from 7/10 to 10/10. From when the ambulance services arrived at her home, over the course of two hours, she had been given large doses of fentanyl, morphine, and multiple doses of anti-vomiting medication. Advice was sought from specialists who recommended several additional therapies including an intravenous infusion of medicine and insertion of a nasogastric tube to decompress Marion's presumed obstruction. These recommendations were discussed, and it was agreed that the nursing team would action the therapies while the physician attended to the many other patients in the ED that day.

Two hours later, the physician was called for further pain management advice with Marion reporting ongoing 10/10 pain. On enquiry they learned that the specialist treatment advice had not yet been actioned. The nurse advised they had been overwhelmed with paperwork and other patient care and had not yet had time to attend to Marion's care. The physician resolved to stop what they were doing and to attend to the treatment themselves. It took approximately one-and-a-half hours to implement the care plan due to complications of obtaining additional intravenous access and successful siting of the nasogastric tube. During that time, the medical review of several sick patients waiting in the ED was delayed whilst the physician attended to Marion's care.

Physician and nursing team initial reflections

From a linear cause and effect perspective, it is easy to deduce that Marion's ongoing suffering was the result of several obvious factors including excessive 'input' of patients to the ED, a delay in 'throughput' with Marion's transfer to a surgical hospital, and delays in 'output' of medical care due to stress, teamwork and prioritisation issues. However, when reflecting on the circumstances that day, the clinicians' 'micro-activity' experiences cast a more nuanced and complicated set of conditions.

The physician had been preoccupied with the care of many other patients since their last review of Marion. Upon receiving the phone call for assistance for further pain management for Marion, they were agitated by the news that the specialist intervention advice had not been implemented, and that the patient remained in severe pain. Seeing the patient again, in profound distress, changed the physician's view on the next 'best steps' and so, despite ongoing need in the ED, they realised that immediate action was required to try to relieve Marion's suffering, and they resolved to do the work themselves. The physician tersely reprimanded the treating nurse for not having actioned care.

The nursing team reported that, on transfer to a short-stay bed awaiting transfer, Marion had fallen asleep and they determined it was better she remain asleep in apparent comfort rather than be roused for additional medical intervention. The treating nurse had decided it was an opportunity to complete a raft of other patient care and finalise admission and transfer paperwork for Marion. In addition, one of the junior nurses needed to perform some observed nasogastric placements as part of her credentialing, and the treating nurse thought the opportunity presented with Marion was ideal for the junior nurse to practise her skills. When attempting to commence the intravenous infusion, the cannula inserted by the ambulance staff had 'tissued' meaning a new cannula was required, but Marion's body habitus made finding a suitable vein by touch and sight improbable and so it would likely need ultrasound guidance.

How then, now, do we make sense of these myriad competing, complementary, and consequential micro-activity decisions? Clearly, the relief of suffering of the patient was foremost in each clinicians' actions, but like so much that unfolds in an ED, the clinical picture varied significantly over time, such that at any one moment what was presented to one clinician varied with what was presented to another.

The physician reflected that, had they known a delay in implementing treatment was a possibility, they would have undertaken the specialist advice at their last review with the goal to ameliorate the future risk of pain escalation and overdosing with opioid medications. Their agitation at learning, two hours later, that the care had not been implemented was a function of their uncertainty about the competence of the treating nurse whose priorities appeared out of order, the ongoing severe suffering the patient, the physician's lack of control over resources to move the patient to the surgical hospital, their own fatigue and growing concern for their clinical decision-making due to cognitive fatigue, and the expected backlog of clinical reviews that would be waiting in the ED upon their return. However, it was the suffering of the patient that trumped all other concerns, and the physician resolved to personally take responsibility for the implementation of the care plan so that they could be sure it was done.

The nursing team reflected that the physician's initial reprimand was misplaced and unjustified in the circumstances in which the task load of the treating nurse had been properly considered and prioritised. The patient arriving asleep and in no obvious distress had supported the treating nurse's decision to delay interventions whilst attending to myriad other important tasks. The opportunity for learning and teaching for junior nursing staff is an implicit and essential task of collegial professional development, and the patient (a retired healthcare worker herself) had earlier consented to the junior nurse practising her skills for credentialing. Upon the patient reporting a return of severe pain, the nurse had followed correct protocols and contacted the treating physician for advice and support.

Whether or not earlier intervention would have changed the course of clinical events cannot be known. Thankfully, the specialist treatment did partly resolve Marion's pain intensity and she was transferred to a surgical hospital where she had emergency surgery to resect nearly 10 cm of small bowel which had become injured from getting twisted in the old abdominal wall hernia site. The patient made a full recovery. This outcome was not known at the time that the clinical team provided care. Instead, the clinical picture evolved in uncertainty over time, requiring repeated reassessments and management changes, as indicators of the patient's condition varied over time.

Insights into Marion's case history based on applying the
ComEntEth model

The following summarises the clinicians' insights as they engaged with
ComEntEth thinking.

Complexity:

- The myriad activities of that day in the ED are justifiably described as
  complex, involving multi-layered interactions between people – networks
  of professionals with different objectives, styles of interaction and competing priorities.
- It is impossible to appreciate the 'whole' of the department. Each of us
  were only able to apprehend the 'whole-part' in closest connection to
  our personal activity.
- The relationships between healthcare practitioners, patients, and external agencies, such as the ambulance service, evolved and changed over
  time and this meant we all had to adjust activities and priorities.
- Some variables, which were not obvious to all of us, affected collective
  behaviour as the clinical picture changed over time.
- It takes a significant amount of time to analyse even one clinical scenario to appreciate the dynamics of its complexity.

Entropy:

- The sensation of 'stress' (raised entropy), ever-present in those of us
  present that day, is aptly described as a function of concern for individual patient welfare, a sense of excess demand, and an inability to match
  personal resources with those demands, together with being fatigued
  and dealing with competing priorities.
- A lack of familiarity with professional scope of practice and practise
  habits amongst staff, together with the lack of experience of staff in
  working together as a team, induced a sense of disconnect between
  many of us, that impacted on planning and prioritising patient care.
- 'Input' demands exceeded any capacity of the ED to maintain a sense of
  control over resources and resulted in reactive forms of action that may
  have increasingly loaded uncertainty (entropic increase) into the clinical picture because the number and quality of the demands exceeded
  rational cognitive apprehension.
- Marion's suffering was very difficult to witness as it appeared unrespon-
  sive to the usual pain management strategies. Many of us felt uncertain
  about what to do next and became increasingly distrustful that there was
  anything we could do to alleviate the patient's suffering.

- The physician felt increasing pressure to find solutions to Marion's suffering and was desperate to have the patient transferred to specialist care for fear she may perforate her bowel and dramatically deteriorate. Their reprimand of their nursing colleague was a discharge of emotional and psychological stress (entropic increase) in response to the distress they were feeling about the ongoing suffering of the patient.

Ethics:

- We each felt an enduring responsibility to care for the people presenting to, and already within, the ED.
- We made assumptions about the motivations of our teammates in terms of clinical priorities, but never doubted the collective intention to try to relieve Marion's terrible suffering.
- Challenges arose in the sense of trust between different clinicians as the clinical picture for Marion changed over time.
- A sense of failure emerged that affected our confidence in our agency to contribute successfully to the relief of Marion's suffering. Some of us feel we withdrew from concern for other patients' wellbeing as we struggled to respond to Marion's distress, and this further exacerbated the ethical distress we felt that day because of our sense that we were not giving everyone the care and attention that was warranted.
- The physician felt badly about their reaction towards their nursing colleague, that they had shown some disrespect to the nurse's professional agency after becoming agitated about the delay in Marion's treatment plan implementation. The physician was keen to speak privately with the nurse they reprimanded to try to repair any ill-will their actions might have caused and to express gratitude for the overall care shown by the nurse towards Marion.

In this scenario, the ComEntEth model makes higher order sense of the array of changing and competing demands and challenges that unfolded in the ED that day. Whilst all that the clinicians identified in terms of the discrete challenges and sensations have been previously described in healthcare literature, our model provides a unified matrix of thinking to coherently interpret how and why these 'variables' cannot be conceived of as independent or controllable. Instead, the attribution of the major attractor – relief of suffering/reduction of entropy – provides an explanation that links the 'micro' dynamics of individuals, professional and personal axiology, and competing priorities, with the success or otherwise of achieving the desirable macro-state of minimisation of entropy of all involved – relief from suffering in the patient and minimising of stress in the clinicians.

In so doing, the interrelationships and contingency of the various agents, their physical environment, personal and professional motivations and vulnerabilities, and the evolution of the clinical picture over time, though dynamic and emergent, can be understood as motivated by an ethical intention to relieve Marion's suffering, whilst at the same time ensuring care and attention for other patients. We can understand how entropy within whole-parts and the broader departmental and resource environment (e.g., the ambulance service) increased over time as energy was expended in trying to realise the best outcome for Marion and others. We can appreciate how the intersubjective entropies related to departmental demand, resource availability and staff shortages became introjected into individual clinicians as their homeostatic mechanisms and internal restorative processes became increasingly overwhelmed. We can see that the clinicians began to suffer and this impacted on their choices as they adapted and responded to their clinical demands.

A change in any one of the key dynamics can be anticipated to have had an effect on the entropic flows experienced within the 'contingent assemblage' of the staff and patients that day in the ED. Whilst the direction of change ('better' or 'worse') cannot always be predicted with certainty in complex systems, any change that did not impede acting in accord with the central attractor of offering relief from suffering, would be supportive of minimising patient and staff entropic production. In contradistinction, adaptations and re-organisation that increase the probability of evolution of the ED away from the major healthcare attractor can be anticipated to introduce high rates of entropy production, instability, and a potential for undesirable macro-state end points.

Framing solutions to the myriad potentialities of the micro-state configurations of the ED, in terms of complexity, entropy, and the ethical imperative of self-other responsibility, promotes optimisation within the self-organising, dynamic and emergent whole-parts (clinicians, patients, managers, operational staff and administrators) whose actions and interactions ultimately give rise to the state of the ED.

Philosophical reflection

We have engaged with abstract, philosophical theorising, in developing our ComEntEth model to illuminate the fundamental organising principles underpinning healthcare. As we reflect on this model, we engage in 'thinking about thinking' or epistemic cognition. As explained in Chapter 1, this form of cognitive processing in Kitchener's three level model, concerns thinking about the nature and structure of reality, our knowing of it, and the role of values (Kitchener, 1983).

In sum, our model proposes that healthcare, as a collective of human activity, or human activity system, is *complex*, self-organising and dynamic. Therefore, healthcare systems have an infinite number of possible states available to them within their phase space. However, healthcare has tended to evolve over time within a smaller set of macro-state possibilities compared to all possible macro-state configurations. Healthcare quickly becomes limited in its expression as a result of the function of 'attractors' on the phase space of its time-evolution.

Healthcare phenomena, as human collectives of activity, are maintained in a functional state because of the flow of *entropy*. Consequently, human collectives, through their dynamic capabilities, seek a position whereby energetic transactions and transformations, or entropic flow can be maximised. In this way, management of entropy functions as one of the cardinal attractors that limit the expression of healthcare within its phase space. Human collectives being comprised of thinking, feeling and acting people, bring a sentient, judgemental or *ethical* response to their circumstances, which further limits expression of the human system to a particular place within its phase space.

We posit that, in principle, complex entities unfold through interactions under the influence of attractors (entropy and ethics) in fractal dimensions. Although we developed our ComEntEth model specifically to better understand healthcare, we realise it expresses three macro organising principles or attractors that prescribe the dynamic unfolding of human collectives more generally. Complex relations, entropic flow and ethical mores can be understood to shape the evolution of all human enterprise. By taking our model to this broader level of abstraction, it becomes permissively inclusive, and we hope, entices others to explore different sites of collectives of human activity.

References

Dunne, J. (1993) *Back to the Rough Ground*. Notre Dame Indiana: University of Notre Dame Press.

Fleetwood, S. (2004) 'The Ontology of Organisation and Management Studies'. Ackroyd, S. and Fleetwood, S. (Eds) *Realist Applications in Organisation and Management Studies*. London: Routledge. Pp. 40–41.

Johannessen, S. O. and Kuhn, L. (2012) 'Introduction: Theorising Complexity in Organisation Studies'. Johannessen, S. O. and Kuhn, L. (Eds) *Complexity in Organisation Studies*. London: Sage.

Kitchener, K. S. (1983) 'Cognition, metacognition and epistemic cognition: A three level model of cognitive processing'. *Human Development*. 26:222–232.

Kuhn, L. (2009) *Adventures in Complexity for Organisations near the Edge of Chaos*. Axminster: Triarchy Press.

Larkin, P. (1988) *Phillip Larkin Collected Poems* (A. Thwaite, Ed). London: Faber and Faber.

Le Plastrier, K. (2019) 'The Entropy of Suffering: An Inquiry into the Consequences of the 4-Hour Rule for the Patient–Doctor Relationship in Australian Public Hospitals'. Doctoral thesis, Western Sydney University.

Morin, E. (2008) *On Complexity* (R. Postel and M. Kelly, Trans). NJ: Hampton Press.

Index

Milton Keynes UK
Ingram Content Group UK Ltd.
UKHW022049141024
449569UK00031B/1559

9 781032 054155